Patient Engagement in Pharma

Sumira Riaz

Patient Engagement in Pharma

A Psychologist Perspective

Springer

Sumira Riaz
London, UK

ISBN 978-3-031-56339-3 ISBN 978-3-031-56340-9 (eBook)
https://doi.org/10.1007/978-3-031-56340-9

This Springer imprint is published by the registered company Springer Nature Switzerland AG
The registered company address is: Gewerbestrasse 11, 6330 Cham, Switzerland

Paper in this product is recyclable.

Preface

Outlining the Current Landscape of Patient Engagement and Psychology/Behaviour Science

Understanding human behaviour and the science associated with the uniqueness of these behaviour enables us to learn how the mind works, how people behave and act and how we engage in decision-making processes when triggered by situations in which the scenarios are positive and negative. I have studied psychology for many years, and I can confidently say I am still learning; this is because of the consistent groundbreaking research entering the scientific platforms, which offers more and more insights into human interaction. Reflecting back on the many decisions and pathways I have been presented with in my career often left me feeling grateful, as each decision led me to learn new skills, techniques and methods of dealing with an unknown situation differently. When building a career as a psychologist, there is no "right" way, and the foundational skills learned are, of course, transferrable to other scenarios present in life. Psychology allows you to learn not only how the brain functions but also how the unique mind of each of us takes what it learns and implements the learning into practice.

We all do things differently, and that is of course okay.

Take a moment to reflect on yourself, how you engage with the world, what information you process from your environment, how this makes you feel, act, and behave. What does your work, social and family environment look like, and what led to this pathway? How do you assess your emotions, what coping strategies have you found useful? Now imagine you are taking care of someone who has been diagnosed with a health condition or whose own health has recently declined. How has this event changed your life and the decisions you make? All these situations and scenarios occur on a day-to-day basis, and people naturally seek information to support them with adaptations. Often, health information is provided by healthcare services, including the pharmaceutical industry. This can include disease awareness campaigns, preventative screening and/or interventional support, and disease information for patients and the public. However, the information can be useful only if people have access to this information, understand the information and are able to implement the learning. Information is of no use if, if not accessible, consistent use of medical jargon and inclusivity are not factored in and if the availability of the information is limited. Similarly, if the information does not align with the individuals' needs, its use is redundant.

This is when psychology can play an important part. The premise of health psychology is based on the theoretical foundations that individual behaviours can be correlated to provide a populational segment to understand how we react to situational events. Health psychologists, merging their knowledge base of human behaviour, behaviour change techniques, interventional development, consultancy and research skills, provide key skills to enable pharmaceutical companies to establish solutions that are beyond just "information". However, understanding not only about information development, the habit formation of healthcare professionals, how doctors interact and engage with patients, and the doctor–patient relationship and communication dynamics offers a deeper layer of how this can be improved to provide a better experience. Referring to the earlier medical model, the introduction of health psychology to the biopsychosocial model enlightens the healthcare field, as it suggested the importance of considering the biological, psychological and social determinants of individuals when making healthcare decisions. It is clear that treating only the biological aspect of illness does not provide a holistic solution; instead, considering psychological needs and social/environmental factors enables doctors to provide more "rounded" solutions. Why is this important? If doctor A provided patient B with a drug and expected that patient B would leave the doctor's office and adhere to the doctor's advice perfectly, this would suggest that humans are rigid and that all follow the same path. Doctor A has not considered patients B's psychological narrative; i.e., Patient B is anxious about swallowing pills, does not believe that drugs are necessary to improve his symptoms and that, beyond the doctor's office, Patient B is struggling financially and does not have the means to pay for his prescription. Doctor A (if based on the medical model) likely did not probe to understand the external situation of Patient B beyond just providing him with a product.

Does this situation sound familiar?

Over the years, I have worked on a number of projects with different pharmaceutical companies. There has been a significant focus on improving patient experience across their disease journey, ensuring that clear and transparent information is made available to patients based on their activation levels and that there is an increase in shared decision making. The pharma industry is aligned with the understanding that its gain is not focused only on sales targets and commercial excellence. Investing in the patient community, working with those who are living with the disease, and developing medicines that are personalised to the patient overall have significant benefits.

This book discusses the different methods of effective patient engagement, not just traditional engagement. In addition, across the chapters, the book discusses a number of elements that will help educate people interested in learning about the structure and process of the pharmaceutical industry, the process of drug development and how patients and the public play a significant part in the development of medicines. The book also discusses health psychology models and behaviour change initiatives. It provides comprehensive but introductory insight into the world of health psychology, models that can be incorporated into patient engagement strategies and case studies to support framing of discussions.

Working as a health psychologist, both in a clinical and commercial setting, has enabled me to provide a 360° perspective on the world of commercial pharma. Sharing my learning will provide the reader with the essential foundations of health psychologists working in pharma.

Acknowledgements

The beginning of this book has been in planning for many years and has been built based on my experience of working in the healthcare industry. I would like to thank all my clients, colleagues and those who I have had the pleasure of collaborating with over the years; without your engagement and interactions, this book would not be possible. I would also like to thank my family, especially Zayaan and Naveed, for the consistent motivation and confidence to complete this project—your encouragement has always been appreciated.

I would like to thank all the staff at Springer, for your support from start to end.

London, UK Sumira Riaz

Contents

Abbreviations

BCT	Behaviour change techniques
Biotech	Biotechnology
COM-B	Capabilities, opportunities, motivation = behaviour model
CSM	Common sense model of illness representation
HCP	Healthcare professionals
PAGs	Patient association groups
Pharma	Pharmaceutical companies
PSP	Patient support programmes

Chapter 1
Understanding the Experiences of a Health Psychologist

Traditionally, a health psychologist is known to work in clinical settings, directly with people experiencing psychological difficulties within a healthcare structure. This is still the premise; however, the foundational knowledge and understanding of human behaviour have driven psychologists into a new field—a professional field when studying psychology is not even considered. An industry that is pivotal in clinical drug development, new discoveries, innovation and reach is endless. This field I am referring to is the healthcare and pharmaceutical industry.

Therefore, what is a psychologist doing work in this environment?

Let Us Start by Understanding the Pharmaceutical Industry

The mechanics of a pharmaceutical industry in the first instance can seem complicated; there are teams within teams, all striving to reach a common goal, be it slightly different. Ultimately, pharmaceutical companies are built on the objective of developing innovative drugs to cure and treat conditions.

The world is dominated by companies developing much-needed treatments, but for these drugs to reach the community, there are a number of significant stages followed by a team of multidisciplinary professionals.

Let me illustrate this in the most simplified terms (Fig. 1.1):

S. Riaz, *Patient Engagement in Pharma*,
https://doi.org/10.1007/978-3-031-56340-9_1

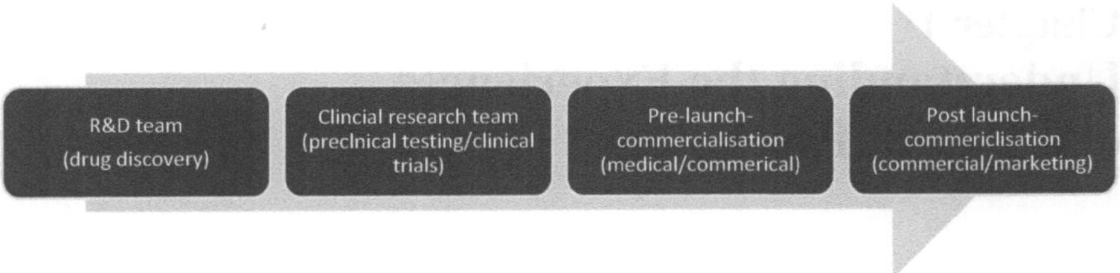

Fig. 1.1 Product development key stages

What Do These Functions Focus On, and What Does It Mean?

If you are new to the world of pharma and the cross-functional system are associated with the lifecycle of drug development, then the following explanation will be useful; however, for those who have worked in pharma or healthcare agencies, this explanation will be familiar.

Function 1: Research and Development Team (Drug Discovery)

One of the first steps in the product lifecycle starts with the research and development team. This team has other sub-teams that have slightly different objectives. Pharma companies are not only focused on developing medicines but also on sourcing and acquiring other companies (namely, smaller biotech companies) that have unique portfolios across rare and complex diseases or innovative medicines, i.e. CAR-T cells and/or gene therapy. To establish these acquisitions, there are teams that exist within Pharma who work by assessing the likelihood of overall commercial gain if a product is acquired or how it fits within the existing portfolio of the company; for example, if company A portfolio (*portfolio means the number of drug/treatment indications aligned to therapy area focus) is 80% across oncology and 10% cardiovascular, 5% nephrology and 5% rare, on assessment, they might not want to acquire another oncology drug, and their focus may be to expand their rare portfolio, so future investments would be focused here. While making this assessment, this team would also consider the competitor landscape by focusing on the future pipeline of other pharma companies. If you wonder how they do this, future pipelines that include drugs currently being tested in phases 1, 2, and 3 are publicly available on the Pharma website.

The other arm of the research and development team is to support the development of new molecules, working closely with scientists across labs to test new investigatory formulas. Once the scope of new molecule development is reached in the early phase, the team works closely with the clinical and research team to start developing an early phase trial (this is not with human participants but with animal models).

Function 2: Clinical Research Team (Preclinical Testing and Clinical Trials)

The clinical research team will focus on leading the testing of the development phase. As mentioned earlier, they work closely with the research and development team to test whether the molecule has any positive results in the disease area for which it is being constructed. Earlier, I mentioned phases 1, 2 and 3 studies. Let me explain these: phase 1: testing with nonhuman subjects; if this has been successful, the trials may move to phase 2: controlled testing, comparing two or more groups, usually a placebo group and an interventional group. The participants were screened specifically based on their clinical history and consented to participate in a controlled trial. There is rigorous testing throughout the trial to measure outcomes. Prior to participant recruitment, research protocols will be submitted and approved before any recruitment can occur to ensure that the trial is safe and appropriately managed. Within the protocol, the researchers will be transparent about the primary and secondary objectives/outcomes of the trial and what they are measuring again. If the trials are successful in phase 2, the test will then progress to phase 3, real-world trials. This basically means that the testing will continue outside of a controlled sample and with a wider populational sample to test the efficacy of the treatment and its applicability. Researchers may also measure the mode of action of the treatment, e.g., IV, self-injection, oral medicine or device usage (inhaler devices, self-injection pens or other invasive devices, if necessary for the treatment).

Function 3: Prelaunch and Commercialisation (Medical and Commercial)

Prelaunch activities can be led by a number of different teams; this basically means that anything that is developed or strategically planned is related to the preparation of the product launch, i.e., the drug/treatment is not yet available to the general public for prescription, and prescribers, i.e., healthcare professionals, do not yet have this option of treatment for their patients. However, awareness of the drug that is preparing to come to market is evident through medical congresses, conference presentations, clinical trial data press releases, publications of efficacy data and potentially plain language lay summaries of trial data being made available to the patient community. Despite this awareness, pharma companies have rules and guidelines that they are required to adhere to and country regulations; therefore, medical affairs teams separate their priorities from those of commercial and marketing teams to ensure that the trial data being published are not biased and are presented to demonstrate the results identified. During prelaunch activities, there are other regulatory submissions that take place; again, this process is country- and regional specific; for example, if launched in the USA, FDA approval is needed, and for European and UK launches, health technology assessments (HTA) are submitted. In addition, market access assessments are initiated to determine the pricing of the product for NHS reimbursement pricing for other health systems. This assessment includes a correlation and comparison of other product pricing. Other assessments, such as economic modelling based on life expectancy, health-related quality of life and other variables, are also completed; these assessments are important for determining if the product is made available to patients.

Function 4: Post-launch Commercialisation (Commercial and Marketing)

Marketing and commercial teams are more involved post-launch, although there is a drive to form a cross-functional team at the launch of a product or brand. At this point, the product is ready to be available and prescribed to patients. Commercial development of brand campaigns with core messaging to elevate the brand's presence in the market (this is especially important when the market is crowded), what would make this product stand out, what would it offer which is different from other existing treatments and is there a core message that aligns with the campaign. With this commercially developed product-specific patient material, including material for healthcare professionals to support them in understanding the product, the efficacy/clinical trial data (if you recall from the early phase 2, 3 trials) are important information that healthcare professionals are eager to access and learn more about the product. The sales teams start leading in-person meetings with healthcare professionals, providing them with information and patient material. At this point, a patient support programme option may also be provided, offering a support initiative beyond the pill. This is dependent on the strategic direction the team decides to take.

As the product starts to enter the market, healthcare professionals start prescribing it, and patients receive treatment. Pharma teams have started to consider real-world evidence research involving studies to measure change in "real world" longitudinal studies over the course of months and/or years. This type of data can be particularly useful if there is a strategic plan to launch in other countries beyond the initial markets; for example, if product X was launched in Europe first and a year later there was a plan for a US launch, then real-world evidence data can be helpful for submission during the FDA approval process.

As mentioned, a cross-functional team is developed around the product, and this team also includes patient advocacy/patient affairs. The objective of this function is to establish relationships (prelaunch and post-launch) to support education and share knowledge and informational support with the patient community in regard to disease management and other means of support. This function helps patients develop long-term relationships with patient advocacy groups and initiate and facilitate patient cocreation/advisory board sessions to understand their disease experience. Establishing these relationships can be beneficial for two reasons: reputational development for pharma companies to illustrate to the patient community that they are taking an interest in supporting them irrespective of any product and understanding the current patient experience in the disease areas to establish a clear benchmark, therefore finding tactical methods to improve the patient experience when the product is launched. Feedback is also an important driver for pharma companies to improve, especially when it comes from their consumers.

Over the past decade, the evolution of the drug development process has been adapted and enhanced to increase its effectiveness and competitiveness. After all, there are many competing pharmaceutical companies working in the same therapy area, with all of their agenda being to become the first to market with the innovative solution, which is going to change the disease paradigm in said therapy area.

The industry is an important contributor to the health system, scientific rigor, and years of testing in a clinical setting before subjecting individuals to testing externally in the real world. There is no doubt about the complicated milestones associated with drug development.

There are different types of pharmaceutical companies, and the internal organisation structure is dependent on the size and therapy portfolio. To put this into context, there is "big" pharma, well-known companies often mentioned in the media, and "smaller" biotech companies, which often have a smaller portfolio and spend time building their brand and reputation in this space. Biotech companies may choose to develop innovations in therapeutic areas where big pharma may not focus on or prioritise topics such as rare diseases and gene therapy. In addition, large pharmaceutical companies may invest in new molecule development or acquire existing modules from smaller biotech companies. Equally, each organisation plays an important role in drug development.

What Are the Differences Between Biotech and Large Pharma Companies? (Table 1.1)

Table 1.1 Differences between biotech and pharma

Biotech	Large pharma
Smaller organisation with less protocols and rigid structure. There is flexibility in the team approach with employees taking on a dual role across the organisations.	Clear structural system across functions and teams with specific guidelines and policies required to adhere to.
Opportunities to be more innovative through scientific investigations.	Focus is often small molecule drug discovery.
May develop partnerships with pharma companies to support with advancements and funding.	Have access to resources and funding across stages of the drug development phase.
May be acquired by larger organisations.	Teams can be affected by organisational structural stages depending on product priorities across the year.

Commercial Value vs Patient Community Success

Finding the balance between commercial value and community gain is not always an easy approach to determine, particularly when pharma is focused on driving product sales and value-cost-based measurements. This is often the dilemma for patient engagement teams working within this organisation; they are often asked to demonstrate value, such as:

- How does this investment translate into an increase in product sales?
- Is the focus an increase in reputational value?

There is a fine line between working directly with the patient community with the objective of growth in sales; this is a compliance nightmare, and the types of metrics and engagements patient teams within pharma are not encouraged by. In a few chapters ahead, I will discuss the types of patient engagement metrics that can be considered when building a patient engagement strategy.

A pivotal part of a psychologist's contribution is their ability to incorporate behaviour change measures into a solution developed for patients. These types of measures can help support the measurement of patient intervention and determine if they are "actually" triggering change. Another area often of interest is understanding the disease journey and the changes that occur across the disease journey if a new product is introduced into the market. There are, of course, other methods with which a psychologist can engage, which will be discussed further. The emphasis here is on highlighting the importance of metrics and success measures that can be considered to be, if not as good as, sales targets (although there are no parallels).

The Spectrum of Patient Engagement

Patient engagement is one of the words you often see together. The initial definition that may come to mind when hearing the words "patient engagement" is based on the following question: why would we need to understand why a patient may or may not engage with their healthcare plan? A patient is an individual diagnosed with a health condition that likely impacts the individual in many different ways, in the short term or long term; therefore, the belief or assumption is that the patient works collaboratively with their doctors to find a solution. We understand from the array of definitions of the term "engagement", referring to the art of connecting consciously, alert, motivated, and communicative. One who is taken in context by conversation or commitment.

When you connect the definition of patient engagement, it makes complete sense that a patient would engage in their healthcare because of the overall beneficial outcomes to them? Right….? Therefore, why has patient engagement potentially become an industry in itself?

First, we need to understand the different layers of patient *engagement—nothing is ever simply.*

Layer 1: Theoretical Connection

In 1970, George Engel and John Romano introduced the biopsychosocial model, pioneering psychiatrists who recognised the limitations of the traditional biomedical model. The biomedical model failed to approach the healthcare system with consideration of the social and psychological impact of disease on an individual. The biopsychosocial model emphasises the three-system approach: (1) biological, (2) medical and (3) social determinants, which all influence and interact. These layers provide a good framework for understanding individual differences in disease management and the considerations that healthcare professionals need to make when treating patients. Prescribing medication and expecting patients to adhere to or even collect their prescription is never a guarantee. Understanding the determinates and circumstances surrounding patients, the family and the social environment provides a holistic perspective; however, consultation times with doctors are often time limited, and having the capacity to spend more time with patients may not always be possible.

Layer 2: The Disconnect in Healthcare and Research

This is one of the reasons why patient engagement has become more central to research, pharmaceutical companies and patients themselves. The society has identified a disconnect between doctors and patients. Health psychologists and theorists have built models and frameworks associated with understanding patient behaviour and engagement, and industry and advocacy have focused on developing solutions to improve this disconnect. Everyone has played a part in the formation of patient engagement. However, patient engagement across industries is still relatively unclear and not yet considered standard practice, although the introduction of patient engagement teams has evolved over the last 3 years. Cavaller-Bellaubi et al. (2021) emphasised a number of calls for action to consider all stakeholders involved in patient engagement, such as (1) the need to identify, develop and share good practices across stakeholders and (2) the need to develop further evidence of improved performance and health outcomes through patient engagement. However, to achieve this, they emphasised the need for culture change (to shift the status quo and drive change to normalise practices associated with patient engagement), clear processes (to drive stakeholder alignment) and resources for stakeholder engagement (enabling them to mobilise resources and budgets towards patient engagement initiatives).

Layer 3: Improved Patient Outcomes

Regardless, collectively, we understand that patient engagement leads to positive clinical outcomes. Good Governance Improvement released a bulletin in 2020 focused on patient engagement, stating that "*there is plenty of evidence to indicate that patient engagement leads to improved health outcomes, focusing on the importance of patient voice, healthcare experiences and preferences, considered crucial*."

The emphasis here is the word "crucial"; understanding how to create a patient engagement framework is crucial, but there is no set method because the stakeholders' objectives who are leading the engagement plans will differ. From my perspective, patient engagement is described in two ways: (1) patient advocacy and (2) strategic patient engagement. Both are important areas that serve different purposes.

There are many different methods by which professionals, patient advocacy groups, healthcare professionals and the healthcare industry engage in patient engagement, and many different workstreams are associated with the inclusivity of patient engagement activities, such as patient and patient advocacy groups, medicine developers, academics, HTA, regulatory authorities, payers, policy makers, market access and research institutions. This can be achieved via a top-down or bottom-down approach. For the purpose of explaining the spectrum of patient engagement, the following descriptions include both high-level "top-down" methods (strategic patient engagement) and direct engagement "bottom-up" approaches (patient advocacy). Engagement preferences will, of course, differ depending on country regulations and internal industry compliance regulations. For example, based on the European regulations pharma can engage with patients for research purposes and patient advocacy groups for non-promotional means. In the USA, the regulations allow for direct patient advertising (TV commercial advertising of medicines) while in Asia, specifically Japan and China, patient engagement is channelled through healthcare professionals instead of directly to patients via industry. This is why it is important to review and understand country legislations when considering engaging with patient groups. Where patient groups are not easily reachable or regulations stipulate methods of engagement that are limited, engaging with healthcare professionals and/or medical societies may be the only method of understanding the patient experience.

Level 4: Patient Engagement in Medical Affairs

Recently, there has been increased interest in patient engagement activities across medical society congresses. Traditionally, a place has focused on healthcare professionals' interaction and engagement, the sharing of research and clinical studies and opportunities for healthcare professionals to engage in learning, networking and developing. The concept of patient engagement across medical congresses is based on the ambition that patients develop initiative. The concept has evolved over the

Table 1.2 Types of patient engagement in congress settings

Congress engagement	Post congress engagement
1. Patient coauthor publication and presentation and elevate the patient narrative of disease experience and engagement	1. Plain language summaries: Production of conference posters/publication by developing lay summaries to share with the patient and PAG community
2. Expert speaker's: Patient experts can present disease experiences, elevating the importance of patients sharing their stories	2. Cocreation and collaboration with patient communities to develop solutions align to the patients/caregivers' unmet needs
3. Congress planning patients are taking an active role in supporting to plan congress activities and creatively on illustrative ways to present research data	3. Knowledge sharing: patient can share information post conference to the wider community

years with the introduction of patient and public partnership research involving patients in early-phase research activities. This aligns with the changes in patient involvement and engagement in their healthcare interactions, and the prevalence of passive to active patients has increased. There are a range of tactical opportunities for medical affairs teams to engage patients and patient groups across congresses and post congresses, as illustrated below (Table 1.2).

I will elaborate on a few examples from the table that have been implemented across industries to put this into context.

Patient Co-authorship

- Producing a publication has traditionally been accepted if it was written by an academic, healthcare professional or researcher. Patient co-authorships across publication development and peer-reviewed articles were not considered a concept until recently. There is still debate and discussion on how to effectively and ethically involve patients in publication development, particularly when manuscripts present clinical research results. The number of patient-authored articles is still limited, but they do exist and are considered "innovations". It is important to assess the type of topic before engaging with patients or patient groups. Similarly, a patient author must follow the International Committee of Medical Journal Editors guidelines expected of all the authors, and transparency on their contributions to the research should be confirmed fairly (Oliver et al. 2022). However, there is a consensus on the beneficial factors associated with involving patients' authors and an overall reminder that the research focus is associated with the patient's story, involving them in telling their story makes sense overall.

Expert Speakers

- People living with the disease are experts; they are experiencing the impact personally on a day-to-day basis; therefore, when considering obtaining an expert opinion, there is no one better who can provide this information than the patient themselves. This is why the drive to engage and encourage patients, caregivers, and family members to attend and present their lived experience across conferences and be part of presentations at congresses is considered very valuable. This communication drives two pathways of engagement: (1) patients sharing their experiences with medical and industry professionals, elevating their needs and preferences across the disease experience and treatment journey, and (2) patients sharing what they have learned from the conference, new innovative medical research, and clinical trial outcomes with their patient community and beyond. Research outcomes and evidence should be moved further into the public domain, and the research reach should be extended.

Plain Language Summaries

- There has been a growing interest in plain language summaries associated with complex scientific studies and clinical research data and the translatable interpretation of the data for lay audiences. Understanding medical research can be challenging, which can then become a barrier to communication and learning. How can people outside of the research field understand important research which can impact them and the frustrations felt by academics and scientists that their research has not been accessed or discussed outside of the "traditional" audience. There are different styles and methods for developing plain language summaries; however, the number of available summaries is often limited. Given that the available guidelines are limited to Lobban et al. (2021), this research study focused on asking patients what information should be included in a plain language summary and other factors. The authors found that the attributes considered "important" for patients were (1) drug approval status, (2) therapy area background, (3) study objective, (4) trial patient population, (5) primary and secondary endpoints, (6) value added to the study and impact, and (7) study limitations. (8) Thank you to the study participants, (9) research sponsor, and (10) author of the plain language summary. In addition, other factors were considered but not important.

Things to Consider When Engaging with Patients for Conferences

Although the prospects of engaging patients across medical affairs conferences sound exciting, there are expectations and guidelines to consider. Local and country regulations are always the first ones, and some countries have strict rules associated with patients involved in medical conferences and transparency in collaborations. Pharmaceutical companies will have their own guidelines and regulations, which need to be adhered to, including contracting with patients, caregivers and/or patient organisations and approving interactions and materials shared with patients. If this first hurdle is successful, there should be some time and commitment to consider good patient engagement. Apostalidis et al. (2015) introduced the patient charter of conference engagement; the principles are still appropriate for 8 years, as outlined below:

1. **Accommodation:** Consider the medical, nutritional and accessibility needs and financial assistance with travel and lodging arrangements as practical. The use of social media and free live streaming should be explored to allow patients unable to travel to participate.
2. **Codesign event planning:** Patients were placed on an equal footing with program creators to help identify core conference themes, select speakers, and evaluate the research.
3. **Education and mentorship:** Patients should be placed on an equal footing with programme creators to help identify core conference themes, select speakers, and evaluate research.
4. **Engagement across the conference:** Meaningful numbers of patients should be included in the audience and speaking roles. Patients invited to attend or speak should be able to attend all sessions open to others attending the conference.

There are other factors and contributions involved in patient engagement in medical affairs; moreover, the push of the term "patient centricity" is more recognised across medical affairs activities.

Types of Patient Engagement Activities Across Pharma and Beyond

Attempting to explain the different layers or types of patient engagement activities is a personal goal of mine. However, I want to be succinct and limit the different approaches. The layers discussed here can be focused on in combination or in isolation.

What Makes Them Different? *Let Me Explain.*

1. ***Strategic patient engagement*** involves developing a plan that effectively aligns with both commercial value and community engagement; however, community engagement is not dependent on the success of the strategic plan. The success of this plan is dependent on the implementation milestones developed by the team (this can be medical affairs, commercial, marketing, clinical research and patient engagement teams), which define the opportunities (others may call it the strategic roadmap). This is often a very high level of knowledge and is specifically aligned with the therapy area of focus. For example, strategic patient engagement plans for rare diseases will differ from those for cardiovascular conditions

because of the competitive landscape in cardiovascular therapies vs the number of rare disease medications available on the market. There are still many unknowns in the rare disease space, with potentially more opportunities in comparison to heritage disease areas where there is an increase in population and more investment in research and understanding. The overall objective of a strategic engagement plan is to identify opportunities, align these opportunities with strategic pillars and provide a clear and transparent method for operationalising teams across industries to deliver on the plan. Chapter 2 will focus on how to develop a patient engagement strategy.

2. ***Patient centricity (referred to as the internal industry pillars of engagement)*** often leads cross-functional teams across industries to find synergies and alignments on how they should be ensuring that patients are at the centre of everyone's thinking. This is the patient-centric narrative initiated across pharmaceutical companies. Interestingly, the majority of the patient-centric vision statements are not dissimilar, emphasising the importance of doing what is "right" for the patient and community, given the belief that ultimately, the business will benefit in the long term. A presentation of the results from a survey involving patients and healthcare professionals across five therapy areas, discussed at a medical affair professional society conference (MAPs) in 2021, suggested three core patient centricity themes, (1) patient impact (patient outcomes, patient empowerment and affordability), (2) patient engagement (understanding patient needs, transparent communication and partnership/collaboration) and (3) innovation for patients (product and service innovation and drug development) within the presentation. There was a comprehensive list of attributes that pharma companies should consider across the three themes, supporting them on their patient centricity mission (Gooljarsingh et al. 2021). PatientView released results from a survey they completed post pandemic, which outlined key factors that patients identified to be important for pharmaceutical companies to be doing to increase patient centricity positioning within the community. There are nine recommendations, but the ones which on assessment, I felt were important to share were as follows: (1) relationship with patient groups: patient groups expect companies to understand the ecosystem of patient groups competently and work in partnership with them, aligning on joint objectives with transparency; (2) development of support services: the survey highlighted that patient groups need to be included in pharma decision making to determine what support services are valued by patients; and (3) patient-centric product development: there was an emphasis on the need to develop personalised treatment, especially during the product development stage, involving patients early, to ensure patient preferences are considered (PatientView 2022).
3. ***Patient engagement in healthcare professions and healthcare systems is*** often referred to as direct doctor–patient engagement and/or access to health services. The feedback method has been utilised within the same setting as patient surveys/focus groups, which hospital and clinical commissioning teams initiate to understand the experience and perspective of patient groups accessing healthcare provision. The premise is that feedback from these groups can help inform

providers and policy leaders on how services can be enhanced and redesigned and what the governance surrounding them is. Research has shown that engaging patients in the delivery or redesign of health can lead to reduced hospital admissions; improved effectiveness, efficiency and quality of health services; improved quality of life; and enhanced quality and accountability of health services (Bombard et al. 2018). Equally, patients have expectations of the health system, namely, value, responsibility, transparency, choice and engagement (Abdelhak 2016). Direct-to-patient care is equally important, and studies have shown that patients with lower activation translate into increased hospital costs, while highly engaged patients with improved control are less likely to make unhealthy choices in regard to their health management (Marzban et al. 2022). Patient engagement within the healthcare system is as important as patient engagement in the community and across industries; each plays a different role, but the overall objective is not as dissimilar.

4. **Research and regulatory:** Over the last year, there has been a strong association between the importance of engaging patients and the quality of evidence provided by regulatory and health technology assessment bodies. Usually, this evidence is required to prove that the research material was co-developed with patient experts or patient groups relevant to the therapy area of interest. Haerry et al. (2018) have developed and published guidance for patient involvement in regulatory processes. These authors emphasise five key values across all guidance: (1) relevance (patient knowledge and experiences are unique and contribute to research); (2) fairness (patients have the same right to contribute to regulatory activities as other stakeholders); (3) equity (patient involvement contributes to equity by understanding the diverse individual needs of patients); (4) legitimacy (patient involvement offers opportunities for patients to be involved in regulatory activities); and (5) capacity building (patient involvement addresses barriers to address involvement and works to build capacity for future collaboration across stakeholders).
5. **Advocacy and community engagement** constitute grassroots implementation. This is direct to patient work, which often has the most significant impact and is translatable to success. Working in collaboration with patient advocacy groups to develop initiatives to close a gap in service and support is instrumental in changing the disease management paradigm. These types of engagement have been increasing since the benefits of engaging patients have been documented. Patient advocacy/organisations structurally differ, and methods of engaging may be flexible because of this. Groups developed for rare diseases are often smaller and are formed by patients or family members themselves; therefore, the capacity to engage may be limited. The EUPATI guidance document provides good definitions of patient types, patient advocates and patient organisations to support planning to work with the community. The authors described "patient advocates" as "*persons who have the insights and experience in supporting a larger population of patients living with a specific disease*" and "patient organisations representatives" as "*person who are mandated to represent and express the collective views of a patient organisation on specific issues or disease area.*" Often,

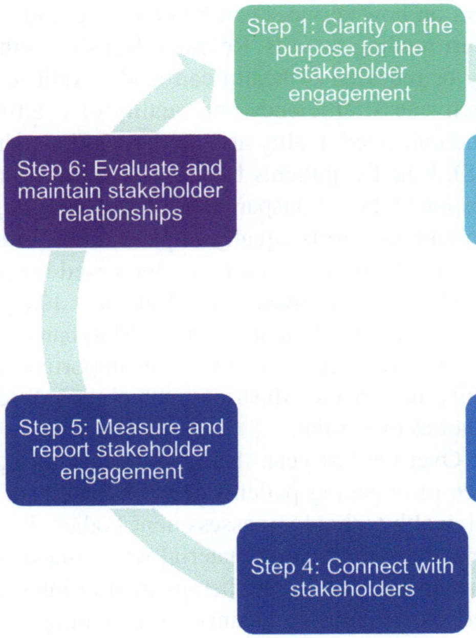

Fig. 1.2 The six-step model is a pragmatic process to consider when initiating PAG engagement

patient organisation representatives are not individuals living with the disease area but rather, in a professional capacity, who elevate the voice of the patients living with the diagnosis.

Working across pharma, I have often been asked if there was a best practice method or model for engaging with patient advocacy groups. Pharma is required to ensure that transparency is provided; however, they also need to factor in compliance and regulations when working with advocacy groups, yet they are truly keen to develop and enhance the working relationship formulated with the advocacy group and vice versa. Ultimately, both groups benefit from the resources and support they can provide, and both groups have a similar objective: to support the enhancement and improvement of the disease journey.

There are many methods of effective engagement and opportunities, and some or most have been developed by professionals working with advocacy groups and pharma on a daily basis. From my perspective and experience, I have formulated a spectrum approach to engagement, as outlined below (Fig. 1.2):

Step 1: Clarity Matters

- Be clear about the purpose of the engagement.
- Prioritise topics that are important for the patient groups.
- Align these priorities to identify joint strategic objectives.
- Development or execution of training specific to patient groups if needed.
- Identify the funding opportunities and processes.

Step 2: Reflect and Key Learning

- Understand what has worked well previously (learn from experience).
- Has there been any challenge identified?
- Are you initiating a new and/or existing partnership with the patient group?
- The diversity of participants included in the interaction is an opportunity to ensure that participation is inclusive and diverse and that factors or adaptations are required to ensure that participation is implemented.
- Internal capacity: Ranking learning using the effort vs impact assessment (high/low effort vs high/low impact to determine level of engagement).

Step 3: Identify Relevant Stakeholders

- Proactivity in identifying patient groups and aligning with the engagement opportunity: Individual and/or group engagement?
- Transparency:
  - What is their role?
  - How can they contribute?
  - What are the number of patient groups you can realistically engage with—considering time and resources?

Step 5: Measure and Report Engagement

- Two-way feedback loop = transparent reporting between both parties.
- Ensure fair acknowledgement of patient groups' time and effort.
- Return to the original KPIs/business objectives for engagement to determine.
- Demonstrate patient vs business value through reporting.

Step 6: Evaluate and Maintain PAG Relationships

- Keep it simple without overcomplicating the evaluating process.
- Areas to consider:
  - Has this engagement added value to the work and relationship?
  - Is it deemed successful by your stakeholder?
  - What difference did it make?
  - Does this engagement result in mutual learning?
  - Has this engagement had a positive impact on the patient community and overall objective?

When Patient Advocacy Engagement May Go Wrong

For pharma, engaging with patient organisation is key. At times, with all relationships, things may divert in a different direction to the intended engagement. I have observed this to happen at the start, middle and end of a project collaboration. Often, the healthcare agency is the "mediator" or the middle team, ensuring that both parties are following the same strategic objective, project timelines are being met, and there is full transparency on the services of support. There are some occasions when patient advocacy groups may become more involved than intended, and pharma may find it challenging to say no to a certain direction concerned that this may impact their relationship with the advocacy group, while at other times, the lack of understanding of roles means that some advocacy groups are not fully aware of how pharma can support them beyond just funding a conference or research project. There are, of course, some patient advocacy organisations that remain fully independent of any funding or collaboration with pharma companies. The reasons for this may be that they feel restricted in what they can say or provide an opinion of the pharma company when funding has been provided. The financial funding provided by pharma companies is publicly available on patient advocacy websites, as outlined in their yearly breakdown. This transparency allows patients, family members and other companies to assess the level of engagement with other companies and where funding has been provided, e.g., through research, conference attendance, patient meetings, etc. McCoy et al. (2017) discussed conflicts of interest for patient advocacy organisations and stated that patient organisations play a significant and influential role in shaping health policy, expanding drug coverage, increasing support for medical research and supporting the approval process. They reviewed more than 104 patient advocacy organisations in the USA and found that at least 83% of those organisations received financial funding from drug, device and biotechnology companies, and 39% of those companies had a current or former industry executive on their governing board. They highlighted an important point relating to the conflicting and competing interests of board members and a lack of evidence to highlight how conflicts of interest among patient groups are managed. The authors recommended that patient groups should provide greater transparency to enable the public, researchers, policymakers, and others to assess the possible conflicts of interest of patient-advocacy organisations when formulating a decision to increase messaging via the patient group. Despite the difficulties in managing this phenomenon, there is a consensus on the beneficial factors associated with effective patient partnerships and the overall positive impact and outcomes of such collaborations with pharma. As mentioned earlier, connecting with advisory groups provides a reach to a wider population, particularly when the pharma client is trying to understand the disease experience from a wider lens, with nontraditional "research participants." It is also important to be mindful that there are a number of patients who do not access or are aware of patient groups; therefore, if there is a research objective to understand experiences with populations who typically are not engaging with advocacy, there are other nontraditional routes, such as community connectively through local centres and services and community and religious groups. This approach is a good method for helping people from diverse populations ensure inclusivity.

How Can a Psychologist Contribute to Patient Engagement?

Psychologists understand behaviour and engagement and how the conscious and unconscious mind influence our decision-making ability and the rationality of circumstances. Psychologists focus on formulating a deeper understanding of the patient's narrative by diving deeper and truly elevating the internalised beliefs, perceptions and experienced people's experiences. This is the description of how a psychologist works in clinical practice.

How Is This Relevant to Patient Engagement—I Hear You Say?

Understanding how people "patiently" choose to engage with their healthcare team is dependent upon and better understood by exploring their internalised system and external environment. Internalised systems focus on people's beliefs, behaviours, perceptions, cognitive schema and externalities, referring to the environment they have been exposed to, i.e., the educational institution growing up, friends, workplaces, relationships, and the country in which they live in the healthcare structure. All of these factors influence an individual's ability to compartmentalise how he or she may react to the given situation. This is why a psychologist's insights and skills in uncovering these inner experiences can be significantly beneficial when working in the patient engagement space.

The insights and experience captured through research are no longer at the "surface level" but go beyond truly uncovering the root cause of disengagement (Table 1.3).

Table 1.3 Examples of attributes associated with disengagement

Individual	Environmental
Socioeconomical statues—including but not limited to financial resources, employment, training, education	Opportunities for participation, i.e., education, healthcare infrastructure
Family experiences: including family system, children, siblings, mental and physical health and illness	Relationship with others, i.e., friends, colleagues, society engagement
Race and ethnicity	Accessing resources: personal, educational and health care information
Personal attributes- identity, motivation, education, confidence/self-esteem, perception, beliefs and values	Earlier experiences: impact/trauma and associations with experiences
Communication: self and others, ability to be expressive	Personality traits: spectrum associated with environment exposure

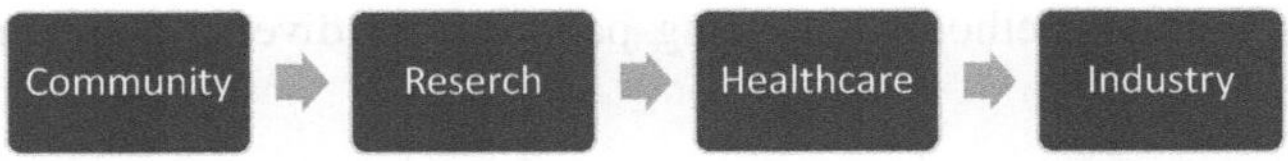

Fig. 1.3 Health psychologists' roles across four domains

How Does a Psychology Partner Contribute to Patient Engagement in Pharma and Beyond?

To explain this in a meaningful manner, I will discuss the role of health psychologists in the four domains outlined in the figure below (Fig. 1.3).

Community

Health psychologists are trained to develop public awareness campaigns and messaging across prevention and policy. In such a role, the focus may be on understanding the links between emotion, behaviour and health-related illnesses; for example, a public health psychologist may be interested in understanding the links between depression and heart disease, socioeconomic determinates and impact on overall health and illness or working with governmental and public health organisations to trigger or contribute to policy change.

Research

A significant part of health psychologist training is based on research skills, from undergrads to professional doctors, and trainee health psychologists embark on a learning journey. Some truly enjoy statistics, while others painfully get through them. With research skills as a foundation, some psychologists stay within this field and develop their careers in academia, teaching or working in a research centre. The research competencies have been helpful, particularly for working across industry roles. Patient research across projects is often built into a project methodology, which includes qualitative and quantitative methods. The types of projects I have worked on include patient surveys, which can focus on understanding patient experience across their journey, treatment preference information, and caregiver/family member experience. The other research methods used can include one-on-one interviews, focus groups, cocreation sessions, and advisory boards; however, the possibilities are endless.

Healthcare

Working within this setting is typically where you see a health psychologist. The role of health psychologists is diverse, but the premise is focused on supporting people in managing their health and illness through psychological interventions, direct support and health promotion, i.e., public awareness. The role has evolved over the years, as has the training. Within the NHS, you might see a health psychologist working in a cancer setting, smoking cessation, obesity clinics and pain management. Taking these transferable learning methods into the pharma industry enables a health psychologist to articulate and include the real and dynamic impact of health and illness while also being equipped with the skills to understand the healthcare system, engage with peers within the system and, importantly, interact and engage with patients and their families in a deep, sensitive, explorative manner.

Industry

On the basis of this book, the number of health psychologists is slowly increasing, yet the dynamics of health psychologists working across projects that are commercially funded (pharma) are still in an early phase; typically, there are limited numbers of health psychologists. Often, you may hear of a role such as that of a behaviour scientist or health psychology specialist. Those working in these types of roles may not be health psychologists who have taken the professional doctorate route (stages 1 and 2); instead, they may have completed a PhD in psychology, research or other related fields.

Over the last few years, behaviour science has taken a positive leap across industry, and the notion of understanding human behaviour and its associated attributes has encouraged pharma companies to further develop bespoke, personalised medication, prevention campaigns, awareness programmes and interventional direct support. These types of initiatives have also been directed to healthcare professionals, as do the days of segmenting healthcare professionals into three types of personas.

The rigidity of such personas has increased into more of a spectrum, as with all behaviour, there are certain high-, mid- and low-ranking traits. Understanding the spectrum of traits and aligning messaging to these traits is likely more effective in the long term.

Nevertheless, there is so much more for this role to evolve and grow, inclusive of opportunities that will ever expand as more health psychologists become aware of other organisations where they can successfully transfer their learned skills.

Challenges and Limitations: Barriers to Effective Integration of Psychology in Pharma

The concept of integrating health psychologists within the pharma industry is relatively new, and to date, there are very limited trained practitioners working within this field. From my personal experience working as a health psychologist, I would say that the field is emerging. There is still learning required from both sides; for psychologists to tap into the skills set, they have learned through training and transferred those skills to develop high-level strategic outcomes in parallel with the pharma industry to see the value of hiring psychologists into their patient engagement teams. When learning and experience are limited, there can be additional barriers to considering supporting the successful transition of a health psychologist working in a healthcare agency across a number of pharmaceutical companies.

Commercial Objective vs Exploratory Planning

Academic research led by a health psychologist is usually related to the individual's interest in a specialism, which he or she would likely explore further through the means of a research project. Similarly, psychologists working across public health organisations build insights and plan interventions through populational data mapping, socioeconomic modelling and understanding of the country's infrastructure. The term "commercial" is not a variable that is considered. Why am I highlighting the term "commercial"? You might wonder, but this is often a dilemma I have experienced or have noted other psychologists moving into the pharma industry have identified. Pharmaceutical companies are businesses built on the infrastructure of drug development, and the drugs/medicines that were once approved are sold to healthcare operations (hospitals, doctors, trusts, etc. NHS), which eventually reach the consumer, also known as the patient. Commercial companies will always have a business objective, and for pharmaceutical companies, this objective will be to sell their treatments across portfolios, increase sales numbers and ensure that physicians are prescribing and patients are adhering to treatment. Whereas a health psychologist is not trained to think and act in this way, a stage 2 professional doctorate includes a consultancy competency that requires a trainee to complete a project as a consultant; however, it does not prepare a psychologist to be commercially aligned. This was a steep learning curve on reflection of my early days in my first healthcare agency. With now-specific guidelines and blueprints to follow, I recall myself questioning what was expected of me in this role. Key things I did not know which I now have insights into (1) always remember the overall business objective, understanding that commercial drivers will help us define the research method; (2) a health psychologist role is still evolving, there is no blueprint, and focus on the core skills you can offer as a psychologist to elevate and support the project; (3) understand and ask questions when others are using business and commercial jargon, a psychologist training does not include this, so there is no expectation of understanding what people are referring to; this is the same for commercial, business-trained individuals, who do not understand psychological terms and models and provide explanations with clear examples in practice; and (4) research is useful and actionable only when it is succinct, clear and what are you trying to articulate in your research finding when presenting these back to the "pharma client". As psychologists, we are always keen to provide all the details, but this approach is not always helpful given the time limitations associated with project deliverables (and people unfortunately do not have the time or capacity to spend discussing findings). Keeping insight presentations to ensure that they are clear and actionable and providing a link to the overall strategy is highly helpful. Pharma clients are looking to you for solutions and insights that will solve their business challenges; therefore, being agile and iterative in your approach is important.

Changes in Connectivity Across Behaviours: Missing Elements

One of the dilemmas I have noticed is that pharma clients do not always know what they want or how to incorporate psychology models and recommendations. However, excitement and engagement are absolutely present because what health psychology brings to the discipline is innovation and difference, a deeper layer of understanding human behaviour and engagement. For pharma, their interest is to focus on their consumers, i.e., patients and physicians, to effectively engage with their consumers. There is a need to fully understand the rationality, decision making, barriers, enablers and overall human interaction while also including the layer of complexity associated with disease experience, prescribing behaviour, habits, norms, cognitive schema and preexisting beliefs of both stakeholders (patients and healthcare professionals); the list of associations and unknowns is endless. There are many different elements involved in understanding human behaviour and psychological profiling. To do this right, utilising a health psychologist is key. However, this is where I believe that pharma is still a "missing element" and that I do not know what we do not know. There is not much information or learning about the effective integration of a psychologist across the product lifecycle or about how consumers profile that the pharma industry has not all made the "link" of how this could and can be useful for them now and in the future.

Articulating the Burden of Disease and Following on Recommendations

The majority of the work I deliver (with the support of the team) across projects initiated with pharma clients is based on my understanding and insights into a particular disease area. Either there are a number of existing insights available or they are very limited. Despite their depth and understanding, pharma clients are always keen to do something different from their competitors, stand out in a crowded landscape and support patients, caregivers and healthcare professionals in parallel across the disease pathway. When working on this type of project, there are certain expectations and integrations needed; no one wants rephrased insights (this means taking already known information through publication and rewriting it using different words so it looks different), the uniqueness of the evidence matters, or how it is interpreted. Alongside this, there is an expectation of clear, strategic recommendations; what can this "team" develop and provide to healthcare professionals and patients to support them? The list of opportunities and tactical recommendations drives the essence of the research. Health psychologists are trained to develop interventions based on gap analysis, but there is a slight disconnect in how this meaning differs between a psychologist and a pharma project. Often, when the disconnect may occur, a health psychologist will dive right into tactical opportunities with the expectation that the pharma client will follow the implementation of these opportunities; however, not all recommendations are followed up despite the emphasis on potential change. I have learned that there is a need to find a medium between what has triggered the interest of the pharma client and what has been recommended by a psychologist and researcher. There is no right answer; the answer often sits where the investment and resources are pushed. As a researcher/psychologist, working with the pharma client to deliver this vision is the goal.

Some key considerations for remembering which summaries this chapter:

1	Patient engagement activities can be inclusive across prelaunch, launch and post-launch stages of the product lifecycle.
2	Aligning and collaborating with patient organisations are significantly beneficial, but there are methods of effective and transparent engagement.
3	Pharmaceutical companies will always have commercial/sales objectives; balancing commercial objectives and community value is important to establish long-term partnerships externally.

References

Abdelhak M (2016) Patient engagement: opportunities and challenges for nursing and health care professionals. Stud Health Technol Inform 225:707–709. PMID: 27332313

Apostalidis K, Ayres S, DeBronkart D et al (2015) Patients included: a charter for conferences. https://patientsincluded.org

Bombard Y, Baker GR, Orlando E, Fancott C, Bhatia P, Casalino S, Onate K, Denis JL, Pomey MP (2018) Engaging patients to improve quality of care: a systematic review. Implement Sci 13(1):98. https://doi.org/10.1186/s13012-018-0784-z. PMID: 30045735; PMCID: PMC6060529

Cavaller-Bellaubi M, Faulkner SD, Teixeira B et al (2021) Sustaining meaningful patient engagement across the lifecycle of medicines: a roadmap for action. Ther Innov Regul Sci 55:936–953. https://doi.org/10.1007/s43441-021-00282-z

Good Clinical Governance. Accessed online: https://www.goodgovernance.org.uk/publications/insights/patient-engagement

Gooljarsingh T, Lee M, Gjurovic AM, Atkins K (2021) Benchmarking patient centricity in pharma across its many stakeholders. Medical affairs professional society conference

Haerry D, Landgraf C, Warner K, Hunter A, Klingmann I, May M, See W (2018) EUPATI and patients in medicines research and development: guidance for patient involvement in regulatory processes. Front Med 5:230. https://doi.org/10.3389/fmed.2018.00230

Lobban D, Gardner J, Matheis R (2021) Plain language summaries of publications of company-sponsored medical research: what key questions do we need to address? Curr Med Res Opin. https://doi.org/10.1080/03007995.2021.1997221

Marzban S, Najafi M, Agolli A, Ashrafi E (2022) Impact of patient engagement on healthcare quality: a scoping review. J Pat Exp 9:23743735221125439. https://doi.org/10.1177/23743735221125439. PMID: 36134145; PMCID: PMC9483965

McCoy MS, Carniol M, Chockley K, Urwin JW, Emanuel EJ, Schmidt H (2017) Conflicts of interest for patient-advocacy organisations. N Engl J Med 376(9):880–885. https://doi.org/10.1056/NEJMsr1610625. PMID: 28249131

Oliver J, Lobban D, Dormer L et al (2022) Hidden in plain sight? Identifying patient-authored publications. Res Involv Engagem 8:12. https://doi.org/10.1186/s40900-022-00346-w

PatientView (2022) Being patient-centric': nine key indicators to define pharmaceutical strategies in 2022

Chapter 2
Building a Patient Engagement Strategy

Thinking Strategically… Is There a Secret Method to Doing This?

What is the strategy? A question is often asked at the start or end of a meeting, irrespective of where the meeting took place, whether it was academic, commercial, clinical research or at home with your family. Identifying a rationale and clear milestones enables those around you to align with the overall vision and develop workstreams to achieve the vision while agreeing on the roles and responsibilities of the "group", which can include colleagues, friends, family or fellow students.

I recall when I started working in the healthcare agency space, a number of acronyms were casually used in meetings, and I was truly lost, unaware and confused. How was I supposed to ask for clarification? Was there an expectation that I should understand what was being discussed? It led me to search for definitions on the internet to further my interpretation, and more importantly, how I was going to approach and solve this. For reference, there are many different methods for "building a strategy" found on the internet, but the best method is your way, finding what works for you and using a variety of techniques.

As a psychologist, you are trained to rationalise problems and assess how you are approaching the problem, i.e., is my decisional process rational or irrational? If irrational, then what is driving the irrationality in reference to the unhealthy assumptions I may be holding about the problem, which is now becoming a barrier? I also refer to this as "clouds", in which the puffy water vapour condenses into tiny water droplets that block your view of the landscape when looking down. The "clouds" can also block your ability to develop a coherent strategic plan and the implementation steps to achieve the vision. Understanding how to move, reshape, and reduce "clouds" from your thought process is important. There is no clear strategy if the strategist's view remains blocked. I am a firm believer that everyone can create a strategic plan; the barrier is the unhealthy narrative, which is often "*am I doing this right*?"

S. Riaz, *Patient Engagement in Pharma*,
https://doi.org/10.1007/978-3-031-56340-9_2

Building a Patient Engagement Strategy

The simplest way to describe a patient engagement strategy is through a plan of action centred on improving the outcomes of patients living with a health condition. For this strategy to be successful, interventions or processes must be developed to close the gap in services/products offered to patients and their families. Therefore, holistically driving positive change.

A patient engagement strategy can take many forms and be led by different stakeholders, e.g., patient groups and healthcare professionals. However, for the purposes of this chapter, the focus will be on developing a patient engagement strategy from the perspective of pharma, including the experience of developing such a strategy with the support of a health psychologist.

Developmental Process… What Do I Have to Do?

There is no right way of doing things, and the premise of this was mentioned earlier; however, there are some flexible rules, if followed, that will ensure that the engagement strategy is built on clear success measures. This is how a psychologist can contribute to forming a solid strategy in comparison to a strategy that holds ideas and loosely formed steps. It is important to remember that patient engagement plans do not have to be ambitious; rather, they just have to be achievable and measurable and capture changes in the patient's environment and experience. I have learned that it is always important to ask yourself one question, "*how will I measure the success of this plan?*", without any measurements; a plan is just a shopping list.

The steps below are specific to a patient engagement strategy developed for a specific disease area and for external stakeholders. There are other types of patient engagement strategies that focus specifically on internal planning across cross-functional divisions, i.e., medical, commercial, clinical, etc. These engagement plans likely differ and work specifically to ensure that teams are prioritising tactics per function without duplicating and learning from each other through these activities. I will discuss this type of strategic patient engagement plan separately (Fig. 2.1).

Step 1: Understand the External and Internal Landscape

- Benchmarking or alignment can help establish what already exists, lessons learned from other companies, best practices in a specific disease area, and patient advocacy group (PAG) analysis, specifically focusing on what PAGs are prioritising in regard to unmet needs.

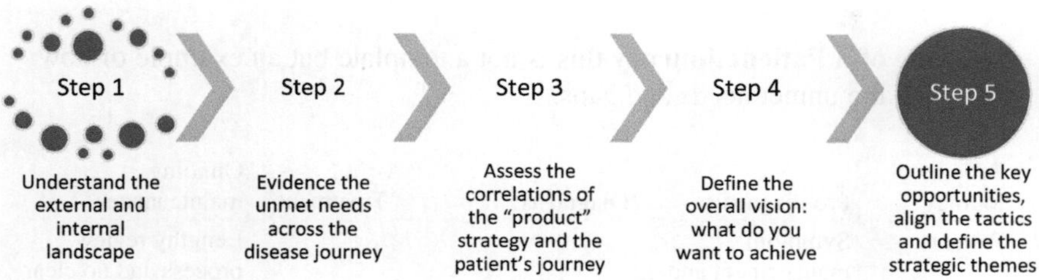

Fig. 2.1 A stepped approach to developing a patient engagement plan for a specific disease population

Competitor landscape	Product/ pipeline	Therapy area expertise	PSP services	PAG relationships
Company A				
Company B				
Company C				

Patient advocacy assessment	Organisational structure	Experience & focus	Capabilities	Policy/ research	Patient support
Advocacy 1					
Advocacy 2					
Advocacy 3					

Step 2: Evidence of Unmet Needs Across the Disease Journey

- What are you trying to solve, and are there clear unmet needs and gaps identified across the patient populations, existing service provision, and treatment availability? As a company, where are your priorities focused across the disease journey?

Step 3: Assess the Correlations Between the "Product" Strategy and the Patient's Journey

- What is your medical and/or commercial strategy for product initiation within the patient journey? Does the patient engagement plan aim to align with the treatment journey? How is this product solving a need? How will this be articulated externally? Are you developing a target product profile (TPP)?

Example of a Patient Journey this is not a template but an example of how to outline the unmet needs and gaps.

Patient journey	Pre-diagnosis	Diagnosis	Treatment	Ongoing maintenance
Patient	Symptom management and delayed diagnosis			Lengthy review process and no clear symptom tracking
Caregiver		Lack of information on interpretation test results		
Healthcare professional			Unclear treatment protocol	

Step 4: Define the Overall Vision: What Do You Want to Achieve?

- Usually, vision statements may be developed at the start or end of treatment. However, from experience, once understanding the disease journey and product strategy, developing the overall patient engagement vision becomes much more visible. Ask yourself: if you initiated the strategy and you were reflecting back on the (hopeful) success of the strategy, what would have made it successful? This reflective exercise can help in outlining what exactly you are wanting to achieve and how your vision should then align with this. Make sure your vision is specific, not fluffy without structure or drive.

Step 5: Outline the Key Opportunities, Align the Tactics and Define the Strategic Themes

- Now that you have your vision, identified unmet needs, product strategy and benchmarking complete. The next step is to assign key opportunities before diving into tactical recommendations. Often people jump right into tactics, without reflecting on the opportunities, what are the opportunities for you as a company, with your product and understanding of the disease journey.

Define the Strategic Themes

- For those who have already built or have viewed a strategy, you will often notice that every opportunity is aligned with a strategy (leverage or pillar). There are probably other words used to describe what this is; I often call it a key theme. Each cluster of opportunities usually follows a "key theme/strategic pillar", allowing the team to prioritise the implementation of the tactics. These themes often remain the same; however, the opportunities and tactics below each theme change over the year. These themes were considered "different roads" leading to the same destination.

To put this into context, I have outlined an example:

Strategic pillar/theme: accelerate early treatment initiation by reducing the timeline of diagnosis in disease A

Opportunity 1
Build and train healthcare professional with diagnostic tools to improve accuracy of diagnosis

- **Tactic 1: Diagnostic tool for disease A**

Opportunity 2
Collaborate with patient advocacy group to develop information about early symptoms/questions and diagnostic testing, what to expect (empower and activate patients) to seek support early

- **Tactic: 2: Patient awareness material: symptom awareness and diagnostic process**

Step 6: Evidence the Success Measures

- As mentioned earlier, no plan is complete without clear measurement, especially when measuring patient engagement is never an easy task. Hence, tactical implementation is important. Each opportunity and tactic proposed in step 6 should likely have a clear measurement embedded to demonstrate success.

Let me demonstrate, if we go back to the example in step 6: tactic was to develop a diagnostic tool to improve the accuracy of diagnosis and informational support delivered via patient groups. To measure the success of this, you can build in short term and long-term success measures:

Short Term

- Pilot sites to implement the diagnostic tool, providing a clear difference between site evaluations and populational comparisons, i.e., pilot site diagnosis timeframe for disease A vs other neighbouring hospital site.

Long Term

- Hospital data and disease journey evaluation to measure the longitudinal difference in the patient's journey (post 12 months of tactical implementation).

What Does a Final Patient Engagement Strategy Look Like?

As mentioned earlier, developing strategies is not something new, but for some, this is unfamiliar (I was one of those people). However, over time and practice, I have learned to develop my own way of creating a patient engagement strategy, which has been trialled and tested in practice with a number of companies I have worked with across pharma. For those who have not seen a patient engagement strategy, I have provided an example of one below; this is a fictional example using the made-up date, but it provides an outline that may be helpful if you might be thinking about creating a patient engagement strategy.

Vision

- The vision statement is focused on the overall ambition/achievement and focus of the plan

Strategic themes	Opportunities	Tactics	Measurements	Timeline
The key pillars which will align to the individual tactics	**Patients**	Disease education in collaboration with PAGs	Website metrics and feedback loop	Q1 (Jan–March)
	Caregivers	Emotional/practical support for caregivers-peer to peer groups	Number of engagements/ attendances	Q2 (April–May)
	HCP	Patient treatment decision tool to use in consultation	HCP feedback (metrics)	Q3 (Aug–Sep)

How Can a Health Psychologist Contribute to a Patient Engagement Strategy for Pharma?

When developing an engagement plan, evidence and insight are important to form a solid direction. Bridging the psychological model to support the strategy provides an additional layer of rigor and direction. However, if you are not trained in identifying psychological models, then you may ask where and how I find the right model that fits with my overall objective and vision. This is why this section of the book will be a helpful guide.

Table 2.1 Health psychology models

Models	Founded by	Focus area
Transtheoretical model	DiClemente et al. (1985)	Patient activation and empowerment
Health belief model	Rosenstock (1974) and revised by Becker in 1974	Rationalise decision making—irrespective of social context
Common sense model of illness representation	Leventhal et al. (1980)	Illness beliefs and perceptions
COM-B	Michie, Stralen and West in 2011	Behaviour change interventions
Theory of planned behaviour & reasoned action	Ajzen and Fishbein in 1975	Social cognition model- focus on attitude and intent
Health locus of control	Rotter in 1966	Social learning theory

Psychological Models…Tell Me More

For those who have dabbled in psychology, they will know there are a number of models, theories and interpretations across a spectrum of psychology. Therefore, for the purposes of this book, the focus will be on health psychology models and which of these can be aligned with a patient engagement strategy (Table 2.1).

Model 1: Transtheoretical Model (Stages of Change Model)

In 1985, DiClemente et al. introduced the change model, which comprises five stages: (1) precontemplation, (2) contemplation, (3) preparation, (4) action and (5) maintenance. The model is not linear but provides a bidirectional flow of how an individual can move from stage one to five. Numerous studies have tested this model and provided both positive and negative constructive criticism. Typically, this model is used for changing behaviours such as smoking cessation, weight management, and preventative interventions. Implementing an intervention per stage is helpful; for stage one, the focus should be to increase awareness and information to support people moving to the contemplation stage. Stage one prioritises supporting people with "readiness to change" (Fig. 2.2).

Example of How This Model Can Be Used in Practice?

To explain the context of this model, an example of when this is operationalised in consideration of a patient engagement strategy would be helpful, especially if you are considering including or wondering how to implement the transtheoretical model.

Fig. 2.2 Stages of change model. (Adapted from Prochaska and DiClemente)

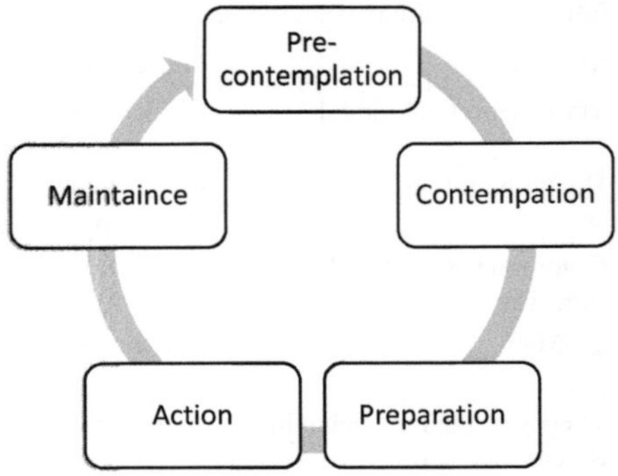

Example 1

- There is a need to develop a patient support solution that is delivered via nurses to activate patients to effectively manage recommended lifestyle changes to support their disease progression.

How to Utilise This Model

The transtheoretical model proposes five stages, as discussed earlier. The goal of the patient solution is to develop a programme that will support patients specifically in managing their weight and diet. A high BMI increases the likelihood of disease progression and impacts the overall quality of life.

Using this model, I propose a number of targeted interventions that are dependent on the activation stage of the patient; below are some examples.

Precontemplation (no recognition that there is a need for change): "My doctor is insisting I make changes to my diet; however, I've been this weight for year and I am fine".

Intervention focus: ***Awareness and informational exchange:*** The focus of this opportunity is to provide basic information to support patients in their readiness to engage in change. People often remain in this stage for a number of months and even years if they do not believe they have the capacity or confidence to make a change or if they understand the value of the behaviour change (cost vs benefits). Providing information and guidance at this stage will enable them to feel informed.

Contemplation (recognising there is a problem and is considering a change): "I am noticing that my weight is increasing my back pain and my ability to complete the recommended exercises my doctors have asked me to do weekly, I think I now need to make a change, but I'm not sure I can do this, as I've tried before."

Intervention: ***Motivational and guidance:*** Here, individuals have started to align with the potential benefit of introducing a change; they have established an inner drive to elicit a change, yet they are "sitting on the fence" with additional support, guidance and motivational messaging that you can support to move patients to the preparation stage.

Preparation (intending to take action in the immediate future): "I've met with my dietician and researched different ways to change my food choices, to help, I have set myself small achievable goals".

Intervention: ***Goal setting and action planning:*** Achievable and smart goal setting provide valuable advice for individuals preparing for action. This timeline can be sensitive if support is not provided to patients, especially if they have decided to change a specific behaviour. Timely and direct support and information will enable patients to feel supported in moving forward.

Action (change is initiated): "I've taken action and introduced made small changes, and I am noticing the difference."

Intervention: Intervention: ***Reward/celebrating milestones:*** Feedback is supportive and continues to engage, especially if individuals have made a behavioural change and are maintaining this change.

Maintenance (adjusting to change and practicing new skills and/or behaviour): "I will continue with my changes and want to learn about other ways to support my weight management goal".

Intervention: ***Information and long-term planning*** to maintain and introduce additional behaviour changes, information and education surrounding the benefits of change are valuable, irrespective of successful change. Once an individual has learned that they are able to maintain a change, instead of becoming static, continuation of this journey will keep people moving toward their goals.

Remember, the transtheoretical model proposes a bidirectional flow in which individuals are likely to move from preparation, action, and preparation to contemplation. When you have in the past decided to make a behaviour change and break an old habit, you are not so easy to do and often our own self-doubt is a key contributor to keeping us in the contemplation stage; alternatively, when we have succeeded in making a change but maintaining the change has been challenging, we may move us back to the preparation stage. Therefore, providing interventional content across all five stages will support patients holistically if you decide to use this model in your activation planning.

Model 2: Health Belief Model (HBM)

Introduced by Rosenstock (1974) and revised by Becker in 1974, the HDM model is a cognitive model that focuses on how individuals rationalise their decisions irrespective of the social context. The HBM indicates that an individual's likelihood of undertaking a health behaviour is influenced by (1) belief in the severity of illness, which may ensure that the behaviour is not undertaken; (2) perceived susceptibility to the illness; (3) benefits and costs or barriers to undertaking the behaviour; and (4) cues to action (internal and external). Self-efficacy, i.e., belief in one's ability to execute a given behaviour, was later included in the works of Bandura in 1977.

To put this content using an example of high cholesterol, the HBM model suggests that a person regularly taking cholesterol medication (a health behaviour) depends on the following:

- Perception of the severity of uncontrolled cholesterol.
- Perception of susceptibility to uncontrolled cholesterol complications.
- Outcomes of weighing the costs (personal and external).
- Self-efficacy and confidence in managing behavioural shifts.
- Cues to action (e.g., awareness of the links between high cholesterol and blood pressure).
- Core beliefs influenced by age, sex, socioeconomic status and other opinions.

There has been ongoing academic discussion on what factors may influence behaviour more; some argue that barriers and susceptibility are the main predictors, while others suggest that barriers, benefits, and severity best predict health behaviours. Interventions developed using the HBM often focus on point four (cue to action), where preventative and awareness information can be developed to trigger individuals to implement a health behaviour, i.e., a negative outcome of smoking, using fear arousal techniques.

Criticism of the HBM suggests that the model does not consider the role of emotions when making decisions and emphasises the rationality of decision making, neglecting an individual's emotional response to the decisional process. The model also proposes a static rather than dynamic approach, suggesting that the beliefs one holds do not change over time; equally, the model neglects the intention to behave only when the behaviour is implemented (Fig. 2.3).

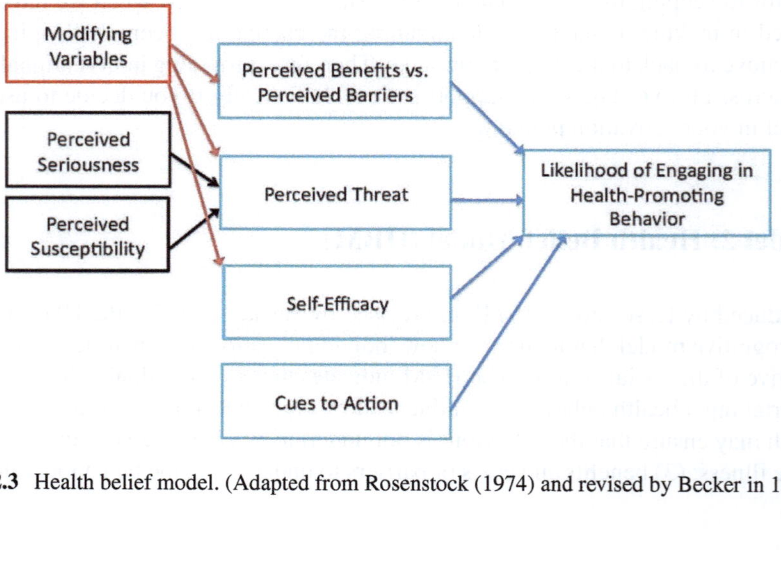

Fig. 2.3 Health belief model. (Adapted from Rosenstock (1974) and revised by Becker in 1974)

Example of How This Model Can Be Used in Practice?

To explain the context of this model, an example of when this is operationalised in consideration of a patient engagement strategy would be helpful, especially if you are considering including or wondering how to implement the Health Belief Model. Notably, the HBM is useful for predicting health beliefs and behaviours and, therefore, formulating interventions. The model itself is not used to design interventions.

Example 2

Company B has recently developed a new diagnostic tool for cervical screening, which will be more accurate than existing methods while providing more efficient results. However, cervical screening use has been considerably low, and there is a need to understand how to activate individuals to attend screening appointments.

How to Utilise This Model

The HBM predicts that individual behaviours are aligned with the core beliefs held; using the model below, the core beliefs are associated with Example 2.

- Susceptibility to illness: "My chances of getting cervical cancer are high".
- The severity of the illness: "Cervical cancer is serious and can be fatal".
- The cost involved in carrying out the behaviour was as follows: "Going for screening will be painful, uncomfortable and embarrassing".
- The benefits associated with carrying out the behaviour are as follows: "Screening will reassure me that I am at low risk of developing cervical cancer".
- Cue to action: Internal: symptoms experienced that are perceived to be related to cervical cancer; external: information read on a cervical cancer awareness poster.

When reviewing the above examples, the main predictor of this model is based on the individual's perception that there is a high chance of cervical cancer, that cancer is a significant threat and that the benefit of screening is high.

To put this into content when developing core messaging for company B, the following recommendation would be suitable:

Domain 1: Susceptibility to Illness

- Core message 1: (a) percentage of cervical cancer patients and (b) number of screening and early detection tools for early diagnosis.

Domain 2: Severity of the Illness

- Core message 2: (a) seriousness of cervical cancer, (b) case studies of late detection (fear arousal response) and early detection (positive reframing), (c) impact of life and future self, and (d) psychoeducation on cervical cancer.

Domain 3: Cost Involved in Carrying Out the Behaviour

- Core message 3: (a) Psychoeducational support/coping strategies to manage embarrassment and self-confidence, (b) normalisation messaging, (c) information on pain management/relief support during the procedure and (d) clarity on what to expect during the screening and questions to ask (empowerment and activation).

Domain 4: Benefits of Carrying Out the Behaviour

- Core message 4: (a) message reframing associated with a real-life example, i.e. another who has screened (b) factual information on the benefits of screening using research and (c) personalisation of screening benefits to individuals.

Domain 5: Cue to Action (External/Internal Events That Trigger a Desire to Elicit a Change)

- Core message 5: External: (a) awareness of screening and (b) local screening locations (accessibility). Internal (a) personal experience of a family/friend with cervical cancer.

Domain 6: Self-Efficacy

- Core message 6: (a) Understanding the screening procedure to increase knowledge and awareness, (b) where to find information to learn more (directional support) and (c) positive framing of the ability to cope with screening (building tolerance of uncomfortable procedures).

Model 3: COM-B Model

Introduced by Michie, Stralen and West in 2011, the COM-B model of behaviour change suggests that to engage in a behaviour (B) at any given moment, an individual must be physically and psychologically capable and have the opportunity to exhibit the behaviour in parallel with their motivations and desire to do so. A more recent model than the others described in this chapter, but the COM-B, which was subsequently developed by Michie and colleagues, provides a behavioural change framework and taxonomy specific to the component in which the behaviour requires change, targeting either psychological or physical capabilities and the subtypes within these domains, which are outlined below:

- Capabilities: subfactors
  - Knowledge, skills and ability to engage in the behaviour
  - The survey included questions about psychological and physical strength
- Opportunities: subfactors
  - Physical, environmental and social opportunities

- Motivation: subfactors
  - Reflective and automatic motivation

Example of How This Model Can Be Used in Practice?

To explain the context of this model, an example of when this is operationalised in consideration of a patient engagement strategy would be helpful, especially if you are considering including or wondering how to implement the COM-B model.

Example 3

Company C would like to understand the current patient experience with a rare paediatric disease to support the clinical trial study and improve recruitment and retention in the trial. However, they would like to consider all stakeholders, including parents and siblings. Currently, research in this area is limited, and Company C would like to develop specific interventions across clinical trial programmes.

How to Utilise This Model

The COM-B is a good model for developing targeted interventions because it provides a taxonomy of behaviour change interventions that can be crafted to specific touchpoints.

Considering the company C requirements, the example below illustrates the use of the COM-B model.

To support the development of the interventional framework, it is necessary to inform the model with evidence and insights to fully understand the experience of the patient group, disease journey, and barriers to and enablers of clinical trial engagement from the perspective of the children and parents/families.

The sources of information can be derived from the literature reviews, focus groups, one-to-one qualitative interviews with children/parents/families, or other sources of relevant information. For the purposes of this example, let us assume that two interviews were completed with ten families (parent and child interviews and 60-min interviews) and that a targeted literature review clarifies the current clinical trial barriers. The discussion guide was developed using the COM-B framework outlined earlier to determine the capabilities, opportunities and motivations involved in clinical trial engagement and retention, and the results outlined below provide a summary captured by the researchers.

A few things should be taken into account when considering paediatric interventions: (1) any intervention should take a family system approach that includes the wider ecosystem of the child and how these interventions interplay across wider determinates; and (2) paediatric physical and psychological health should be integrated, and targeting should focus on the impact and burden of each intervention (Table 2.2).

Table 2.2 COM-B examples

COM-B	Subfactors	Example insights	BCT[a]
Capabilities	Psychological	Lack of child friendly or accessible clinical trial information for parents/HCPS to share and discuss with children	Education
	Physical *(strength and stamina)*	Participating in tests and measurements on a weekly basis is burdensome for the family system Parents expressed a lack of knowledge on how to access information about clinical trials and did not feel confident in the decision-making process Clinical trial information is often complicated and difficult to comprehend	Enablement Instructions on how to perform a behaviour Pharmacology support
Opportunities	Physical	Difficulties travelling to trial centres as they are not at local reach, with other children, the capacity to attend a centre every week will be difficult.	Social and environmental support
	Social	When taking to other families who have previously participated in clinical trials, the feedback has been varied (positive and negative) which is influencing our decision. There is not an internal consensus between our family that participating in the trial is the right thing to do.	Social support (practical & emotional)
Motivation	Reflective	Lack of decision aid support during recruitment and information about trials Low confidence in effectively participating in trial and no clarity on support provided Lack of understanding of "role" of parent/ patient in the trial	Demonstration of behaviour Credible source
	Automatic	Anxious about the tests and investigation required Frustrated with the lack of clarity Concerned that the decision to enrol my child who may not be able to cope	Information about health consequences Problem solving Credible source

[a]Behaviour change taxonomy (Michie et al. 2011)

Model 4: Common Sense Model of Illness Representation (CSM)

Introduced by Leventhal et al. in 1980 and adapted by Lau and Hartman in 1983, a social cognitive model has the premise that when an individual is presented with a threat, they form a cognitive and emotional representation of that threat. The model provides a perspective on how people may perceive, interpret and respond to health- or disease-related information. This model emphasises the interpretation and consideration of lay beliefs and/or the presentation of health treatments. We know through health psychology theories that individual core beliefs play a central role in motivating individuals' decisions to engage in treatment or to find methods to help them cope with illness treatment; moreover, if individuals are irrational and unhelpful, they can then engage in seeking treatment and support, therefore acting as a barrier.

The CSM model suggests that facilitating a comprehensive understanding of patients' beliefs and how these impact treatment decisions is fundamental to informing the types of interventions that may be introduced to effectively support adaptive or change maladaptive behaviours in the short and long term.

The model proposes two types of beliefs: (1) a cognitive representation of the illness formed by information recall (earlier experiences or other experiences of illness) and (2) emotions that operate and interact together when coping responses are formed.

To support emphasis on the important aspects of the model, the following are the key considerations and model attributes:

The five distinct cognitive dimensions are interrelated:

1. Cause—*beliefs associated with the "cause" of the illness*
2. Consequences—*beliefs associated with the "impact" of the illness on life*
3. Identity—*the symptoms/label applied to the illness/condition*
4. Personal control—*belief that the illness/condition can be cured/controlled by personal actions*
5. Timeline—*the expected duration/time of the illness and/or symptom*

The CSM model indicates that illness representations are schematic in nature and are activated upon presentation of specific illness stimuli (i.e., earlier experience or posters at the doctor's office). When this is activated, coping methods that have been learned and associated with this illness belief are equally activated alongside the representation (Fig. 2.4).

Example of How This Model Can Be Used in Practice?

To explain the context of this model, an example of when this is operationalised in consideration of a patient engagement strategy would be helpful, especially if you are considering including or wondering how to implement the common-sense model of illness representation.

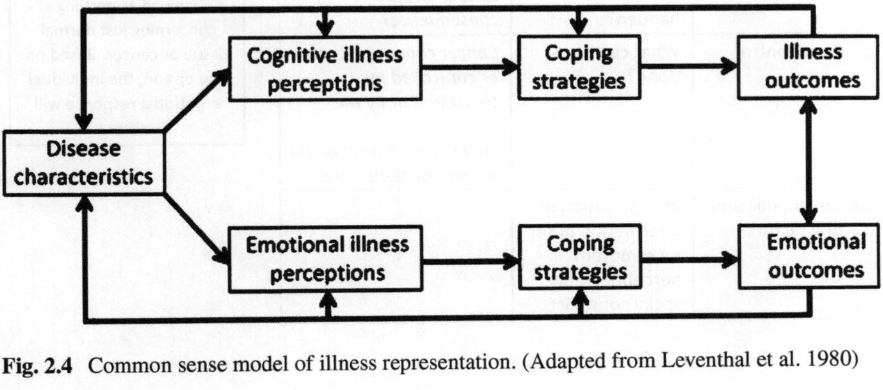

Fig. 2.4 Common sense model of illness representation. (Adapted from Leventhal et al. 1980)

Example 4

Company D has just acquired a new drug in oncology, and individuals diagnosed with and living with cancer have negative health and emotional outcomes. Patients are interested in understanding the psychosocial determinants of illness representations and coping strategies currently applied by patients. This information will enable them to provide appropriate support to patients and design patient material and messages.

How to Utilise This Model

To inform a 360° view of the current landscape and patient experience, the model requires information to formulate a populational understanding. Types of information that can be useful include published research via a targeted literature review and qualitative and/or qualitative research of patients (one-to-one/focus groups/surveys). The model can be used to develop discussion guides or surveys for research, and using the constructs of the model to formulate the research material will ensure that the insights captured are relevant to the overall outcome of the project. Below is an example of how the model can be used for the analysis of data.

CSM- *cognitive*	Constructs	Insight narratives
a. Identity	What is it?	*I think I have cancer (noticed a lump)*
b. Cause	Why did it happen?	*My uncle has cancer, it's in the family or I have caused this by my lifestyle choices* *I know cancer causes pain*
c. Timeline	How long will it last?	*Cancer will be in my life for a long time and is likely to recur*
d. Consequences	What will happen?	*Cancer will trigger serious health consequences*
e. Cure/control	What can be done?	*Cancer cannot be cured or controlled by treatment or by me* *Taking medication might relieve my symptoms*
Socioeconomic and cultural factors	Interpretation of information based on symptom perception and social construct	

Emotional representation

Identified symptom will trigger an emotional response this will differ depending on how the individual assess the symptoms, i.e., lump under the arm might be viewed as nothing concerning just normal tissue or cancer. Based on the option, the individual emotional response will differ.

Coping Response (Approach or Avoidant) and Interventional Approach

The CSM predicts that negative cognitive representations, along with negative emotional representations, lead to more negative illness perceptions. Identifying the specific relationship between a patient's illness perceptions at one point in time, how they change over time and future beliefs can support the identification and development of appropriate interventions for cancer patients. Interventions that target specific illness perceptions are recommended to reduce the likelihood of maladaptive coping and poor psychological health in the future.

Model 5: Theory of Planned Behaviour (TPB) and Reasoned Action

The TPB model is often referred to as the social cognition model. The premise of the model is focused on the role of attitude in behaviour and emphasises on the notion of "intention" when undertaking a health behaviour. Introduced by Ajzen and Fishbein in 1975, the model suggests that intentions can be modified by the perceptions and attitudes of an individual, and the individual's perceived control of that health behaviour and the individual's perceived benefit and cost of the behaviour.

Based on the model, the TPB predicts that after taking into account the internal and external factors, people will intend to undertake a health behaviour, for example, healthy eating, if they or their significant other/family/friends believe it to be beneficial (subjective norm) and they perceive themselves as having the capabilities and capacity to do it (learnt from past experiences/perceived behaviour control refers to one's belief that they have control).

The model has criticisms, one of which is applied because of its lack of a directional component; however, it has been recognised as a good model for predicting the intention of behaviour across a number of preventative campaigns (Fig. 2.5).

Model 6: Health Locus of Control

Originating from the work of Rotter in 1966, the health locus of control model is based on social learning theory and attribute theory. Social learning theory proposes that individuals have a generalised expectancy of the outcome of their actions when the outcome is dependent on their earlier experiences and the extent to which the outcome is favourable or valued. Individuals either feel that they have control over their behaviour and the outcome of this behaviour on their life or that the external environment plays a significant part in controlling the outcome. The attribute theory proposes four distinct factors: (1) internal or external, (2) specific or global, (3) controllable or uncontrollable, and (4) stable or unstable.

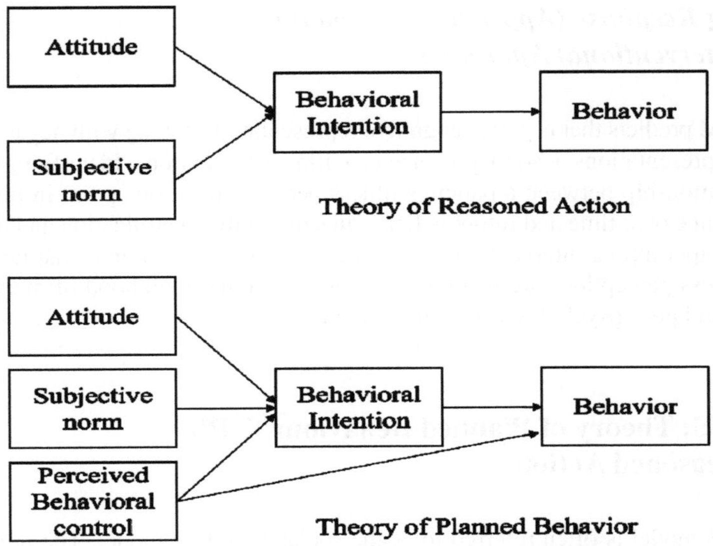

Fig. 2.5 Theory of planned behaviour and reasoned action. (Adapted from Ajzen and Fishbein 1975)

The external "chance" attributes might include "It's a matter of luck whether I get complications", which are less likely to lead to health behaviours than external "powerful" attributes such as "the doctor will tell me what to do for the best".

Criticism for the model suggests that the internal locus of control indicates a greater burden on self-responsibility, with the potential to trigger psychologically ill health.

Why Is This Important?

As discussed, to target and measure change, there is a need to identify and target behaviour change. The fictional examples I have outlined and discussed within the chapter are examples of when a health psychologist can be utilised to fully form a structured engagement strategy using these models as a foundation. By aligning interventions with specific constructs, one will be able to measure the specific change, instead of being loosely proposed without any real focus. Therefore, developing a holistic and robust engagement strategy for all stakeholders (patients, families, caregivers and healthcare professionals) is desirable.

References

Ajzen I, Fishbein M (1975) A Bayesian analysis of attribution processes. Psychol Bull 82(2):261

DiClemente CC, Prochaska JO, Gibertini M (1985) Self-efficacy and the stages of self-change of smoking. Cogn Ther Res 9:181–200

Leventhal H, Meyer D, Nerenz DR (1980) The common sense representation of illness danger. In S. Rachman (Ed.), Contributions to medical psychology (Vol. 2, pp. 17–30). New York, NY: Pargamon

Michie S, van Stralen MM, West R (2011) The behaviour change wheel: a new method for characterising and designing behaviour change interventions. Implement Sci 6:42. https://doi.org/10.1186/1748-5908-6-42. PMID: 21513547; PMCID: PMC3096582

Rosenstock IM (1974) The health belief model and preventive health behavior. Health Educ Monogr 2(4):354–386

Chapter 3
Implementation Science

How Can Patients Be Activated to Engage with Their Healthcare? What Is Shared Decision Making?

Over the past few years, there have been a number of articles and discussions at patient engagement conferences about the concept of shared decision making (SDM). The definition of this variable varies depending on the audience to which it is presented. However, shared decision making is and has been a concept regarded in health psychology as the essence of effective doctor–patient communication in parallel with patient empowerment (improving self-efficacy). The National Institution of Healthcare and Excellence (NICE) defines shared decision making as *"a process in which healthcare professional works together with a person to reach a decision about care, based on the individual preferences, beliefs and values."*

I often reflect on what is considered the main premise of effective shared decision making and consider the points below to be logical;

- **Collaborative** discussion between healthcare professional and the individual.
- **Transparent** information that is understandable and evidence-based to support the individual in making an **informed decision** (*the word "informed" is important to highlight here, and the individual should be provided with enough information to feel confident that they have been able to make a balanced decision*).
- **Empower and activate** individuals to feel part of the consultation process; they are not being told; they are being consulted with.

In this chapter, I will provide a framework for understanding and developing shared decision-making opportunities and how this can be implemented in practice. Working with a number of pharmaceutical companies, on reflection, I have learned that the concept of SDM is still relatively new, irrespective of the ongoing discussions externally. Pharma is only beginning to develop tactics associated with implementing shared decision making, and the methodologies offered to them vary from

S. Riaz, *Patient Engagement in Pharma*,
https://doi.org/10.1007/978-3-031-56340-9_3

agency to agency. The approach I will discuss is based on health psychology principles and my own experience developing such initiatives. However, there is an overall consensus that knowledge and awareness among both professionals and patients, as well as tools and training, are needed for SDM to be widely implemented. Despite these efforts, there is still a need to move beyond the standard concept of SDM to determine how to further develop this approach to become the norm of engagement.

The framework discussed below can be applied to any therapy area; it provides an overarching model of effective shared decision making across four main concepts: (1) collaboration, (2) transparency, (3) informed choice/decision and (4) empowerment and activation. Each concept includes sub-attributes that should be considered. I will discuss each concept individually.

Concept 1: Collaboration

Communication

Guideline 1

- Good doctor–patient communication is essential for health promotion, disease prevention and collaborative discussion.

How Can This Be Addressed?

- Recall a time when you have been at a doctor's appointment, after waiting 30 minutes for your appointment (even though you were on time), you walk in and your doctor is facing the computer screen, head down and asks, "*what brings you here today?*". As an individual walking into that situation, you might assume that you are on a timer and should efficiently verbalise your symptoms and quickly depart; if possible, —would you leave feeling like you have had a valuable conversation with your doctors? Most likely, not.

This is why good communication enables patients to share information about their health, symptoms, and the impact this communication has on their quality of life. The premise is for healthcare professionals and patients to have a mutual discussion where shared knowledge is appreciated, information is analysed and treatment and care are decided collaboratively. From experience, I have observed that good communication builds a stable foundation for future interactions and relationship building. This is a similar method psychologists consider when working with patients therapeutically, described as the "therapeutic relationship".

Often, relationship breakdown occurs when communication is misinterpreted, the consultation feels rushed, the information shared is not fully understood by the patient and vice versa, and the healthcare professional has not aimed to understand the actual concerns identified by the patients. This misinterpretation and its impact on the overall health outcomes of a patient can be detrimental. Hence, understanding how pharma can support patient and doctor communication through engagement, training, and interventional support is important.

Within the health psychology field, the concept of doctor–patient communication is not new; it has been emphasised for many decades, and to conceptualise the types of doctor–patient subtypes, we first need to outline the profiles and perspectives to enable us to dive deeper, as outlined below.

- *The deviated patient's perspective*
  - The belief was that patients often mask their real symptoms, and the role of the doctor was to uncover what the real issues were.
- Authoritarian doctor perspective or patient-centred approach
  - Traditionally, authoritarian doctors' styles were described as rigid, focusing primarily on the doctor leading the conversation by sharing his/her skills and knowledge of medicine. While this method may be appreciated by some individuals, others prefer a patient-centred style.
  - A patient-centred style of communication places patients in focus, and doctors spend time asking patients to share their experience and knowledge of the symptoms experienced while they demonstrate interpersonal skills, such as reflective and active listening.
- The interactive dyad perspective
  - This approach is dynamic and illustrates a shift in doctor–patient communication. Both stakeholders communicated with consideration of cultural sensitivity and individual differences, simplifying language to ensure that there was a consensus of understanding among the interactions.

What Does This Mean for Pharma?

Over the last few years, with emphasis on all solutions, particularly when pharma teams are trying to establish an accurate understanding of habitual doctor–patient behaviour and response, there has always been a need to improve this interaction to ensure that the discussions are correlated with the interactive dyad approach and patient centred. The question I am often asked about is what types of recommendations or techniques should be included in the materials to support improving this engagement.

Lucky for you, I do have some suggestions that have been trialled and tested across a number of projects I have worked on with a range of pharma companies, as outlined below.

Effective communication between a patient and doctor should include consensus and opportunity;

- Explore the disease and symptomatic behaviour
- Explore the holistic impact of disease on patients/demonstrations interest in the overall burden, i.e., work, family, etc.
- Discussion and alignment of treatment plans
- Inclusion of preventative and health information
- Characteristics of a therapeutic interaction (compassion, self-awareness)
- Consensus of expectations from both sides (doctor and patient)

Research has often demonstrated the benefits of a patient-centred approach, such as overall patient satisfaction and increased adherence to treatment initiated by a doctor (Edgman-Levitan and Schoenbaum 2021).

Concept 2: Transparency

Informational Transparency

Guideline 2

- The information provided to individuals should be clear, understandable, accurate and readable, taking into consideration their health literacy abilities.

How Can This Be Addressed?

- Health literacy is often described as the application of cognitive skills, and this definition has evolved over time, leading to it being described as a function that enables individuals to improve their health by making informed decisions, increasing control and taking responsibility for their health.
- Nutbeam (2000) proposed a three-level health literacy concept that included the following:
  - ***Level 1: Functional Health Literacy***
    Basic reading and writing skills help individuals function in their healthcare journey.
  - ***Level 2: Interactive Health Literacy***
    The development of personal, cognitive and literacy skills can improve individuals' capacity to act independently based on the knowledge learned by applying the information.
  - ***Level 3: Critical Health Literacy***
    Advanced cognitive skills and the ability to critically evaluate and utilise information to actively participate in health initiatives and discussions and to have control over personal health decisions.

Why Is Health Literacy Important?

A number of studies have correlated the prevalence of limited health literacy with the overall impact on health; individuals with low health literacy have poorer overall health, are less likely to access preventative screenings, have delayed responses to medical interventions, and have overall lower adherence to treatment (Paasche-Orlow et al. 2005; DeWalt et al. 2004). With this knowledge and considering that individual health literacy likely impacts individuals' ability to engage with treatment plans, there is a significant need to change how information is formulated.

You might be thinking, there is always a framework or model insisting that change is important, despite theoretical frameworks such as the one discussed above. In Jordon et al. directly asked patients what they perceived to be important attributes of health literacy. The results were interesting; hence, I am interested in sharing these findings with you. The study showed that patients felt that there were key attributes that needed to be considered to support health literacy, such as the following:

1. Knowing *when* to seek health information
2. Knowing *where* to seek health information
3. Verbal communication skills (being able to adequately describe health issues and understand the response provided to them by their healthcare professional)
4. Retaining and processing information (understanding the information shared with them by their doctor)
5. Assertiveness
6. Application skills (following instructions and implementing procedures)

How Can You Measure Health Literacy?

There is currently no single specific measure of health literacy; there are a number of different types of questions that can be used to assess health literacy. If you decide to go down the cognitive functioning route as cognition weights highly, as described in the Nutbeam (2009) model, then a method such as readability scores, word recognition, comprehension and numeracy skills is used. Other ways to assess health information include developing specific health-related questionnaires that individuals can complete to determine their level of efficacy and understanding of the information presented to them, i.e., multiple-choice questions such as knowledge about symptoms, cause, self-management and ability to implement the health advice provided to them by their healthcare professional.

There is also an opportunity to develop screening questions that can be incorporated into patient support solutions. These questions will likely be self-reported options, bespoke to the disease area.

Incorporating a cognitive and self-report questionnaire will ensure that individuals' health literacy will cover cognitive (does this individual understand the information provided to them) and self-efficacy (is this individual confident in providing health information). This twofold method ensures that the measure is holistic and factored in the overall functionality of an individual.

What Does This Mean for Pharma?

Consequently, a better understanding of people's health literacy is crucial for adapting health-related information, services and designing successful health education programs. Pharma vision statements are often related to being patient-centric, including the solutions they develop for their key stakeholders (people living with the disease). It just does not make any sense if patient material and content are being developed and not effectively utilised as they were intended to do so. If pharma companies are concerned that patients are not acting on the health information/advice being offered to them by the various interventions, awareness campaigns and doctor consultations, then maybe it is time to consider that the patient population they are targeting requires a bespoke, tailored solution based on their health literacy ability and action.

Concept 3: Informed Choice

Guideline 3

Information should be balanced and fair to enable informed choice.

What defines "informed choice"? Well, this depends on the premise this is sought. Marteau et al. (2001), and the General Medical Council (1999), define informed choice as "*one that is informed, consistent with the decision makers' value and behaviourally implemented.*" Interestingly, the GMC (1999) continues to describe "informed decision", which is "*one where a reasoned choice is made by a reasonable individual using relevant information about the advantages and disadvantages of all possible course of action, in accordance with the individual's belief.*"

Within health psychology, informed choice and informed decision-making relate to the ability of an individual to rationalise a decision using methods such as pro- and cons and personal preferences for the decision while taking a balanced perspective if there is available literature or information to support their thinking. As mentioned earlier, feeling part of the decisional process triggers attributes associated with empowerment and activation.

What Does This Actually Look Like in Practice?

To support individuals in making informed choices, there is a need to provide accurate and accessible information that incorporates a balanced view (benefits and costs). There are numerous concepts that outline the process of informed choice for research participation, and I believe the same principles apply here.

Pharma clients often discuss the benefits of decision aids (a tool/material provided to healthcare professionals for use with their patients to enable informed choice about a specific decision, i.e., treatment, diagnostic tests, screening, etc.) and how this type of tool can be utilised to provide clear and transparent information to patients and support their informed choice. Often, they ask if there is evidence that outlines the benefits of a decision aid, preferably trialled and tested. In 2017, Stacy and colleagues completed a comprehensive systematic review that assessed the overall outcomes and effects of using a decision aid tool. The review suggested that, compared to usual care, decision aids reduce the proportion of undecided participants and have an overall positive effect on patient-clinical communication. Patient satisfaction associated with choice and the overall process of making a decision were also greater in these patients than in those receiving usual care.

Overall, there is a consensus that to enable informed choice and informed decision, people will feel more knowledgeable, better informed and confidently make a choice that aligns with their personal values with a more accurate risk perception.

Concept 4: Empower and Activation

Guideline 4

Individuals feel in control and have the opportunity and self-efficacy to take action.

The buzz word I often hear in pharma and across agencies is empowerment and activation. The concept of patient engagement sits within the realms of supporting people and developing interventions to lead to empowerment and activation. Kim and Lee (2016) describe psychological empowerment as *"intrinsic task motivation reflecting a sense of self control in relation and an active involvement with one's role"*. Empowerment is recognised globally across world health organisations and health agencies as the core concept in achieving and elevating individuals' voices to be able to commit to feeling part of the system, of self and community, and identifying and facilitating decisions, especially when these decisions are centred around the individual.

Therefore, how does it feel to be activated and empowered? Well, it will most definitely differ for many; experience itself is individualised, and considerations of community, culture, and socioeconomic status may contribute to how one feels when they are activated. For example, people might come across someone who is highly empowered and activated; however, the ecosystem surrounding them does not offer the opportunities or facilities they require to take action, and vice versa—the inner drive may be there, but there is no external buffer to continue this. This is often the case across healthcare services, and opportunities for patients to feel empowered may not always be forthcoming. Cyril et al. (2016) suggested that there is still capacity to improve knowledge about the role of empowerment in communities and capacity building for overall health promotion. For the scope of this discussion, I am referring to individualised empowerment; however, I would note that there are two variations of interventions for increasing empowerment: (1) populational/community empowerment and activation, usually taking a top-down approach with the aim of changing behaviours across communities, i.e., health promotion campaigns, and (2) individual/self-empowerment and activation, which are designed to focus on individual/personal outcomes.

What Does This Actually Look Like in Practice?

In practice, I would take the opposite definition of empowerment and activation and use this as a guiding tool to indicate how best to support patients to feel the opposite. Let's take this method: across healthcare, patients are often still not included in decisions about their overall care, which leads to feeling disempowered, interpreted as "feeling less powerful or confident." The opposite of this approach would be to provide people with a platform to feel "power and autonomy to make decisions about their own care." The overall goal of programmes developed to increase empowerment is to decrease inequalities in health and health outcomes. The term I would like to use here is "autonomy." Bandura's social cognition theory emphasises the importance of self-efficacy (confidence in oneself to carry out a behaviour change, stay motivated and have influence over their personal environment). The model suggests that the three factors that influence the self-system are (1) persons' attitudes, (2) abilities and (2) cognitive skills.

Based on Bandura's model, the four methods of increasing self-efficacy are as follows:

(a) ***Mastery Experience:*** learning and implementing the learned skills, the concept of practice and the availability of opportunities to practice.

Action Developing opportunities for patients to practice skills to lead discussions with their healthcare team, consultation guides and discussion prompts support the notion of mastering the skills, hence increasing self-efficacy.

(b) ***Social Modelling:*** Social observation or seeing others complete a task or behaviour shift can influence an individual's desire to do the same, increasing their belief that they do have the capability to do so.

Action Peer-to-peer stories can be beneficial for inclusion across messaging and content. Stories of others who have achieved the behaviour shift and the benefits they have noticed.

(c) ***Social Persuasion:*** The premise of this, as Bandura suggested, is based on the art of persuasion. He believed that people can be "nudged, persuaded" to believe in themselves, triggering them to feel that they have the skills and capabilities to fulfil the action. The persuasion often aligns with building confidence in others through complements and encouragement, i.e., *"I believe in you; you can do this."*

Action Developing messaging or content using positive message framing, which offers encouragement and achievable actions to build self-efficacy.

(d) ***Psychological response:*** Bandura states that emotional and physical reactions are not important; rather, they indicate how an individual perceives and interprets this intensity of emotion. How we respond to a situation or build up our internalised belief about the situation can influence our self-efficacy. For example, if you are nervous about starting a conversation with your doctor about your treatment, you may develop a weak sense of self-efficacy about this situation, which will keep you from speaking to your doctor.

Action Providing emotional well-being support to identify the "activating trigger" and the emotional response aligned with that event will help reduce the unhelpful belief associated with it and support the improvement of self-efficacy in that given situation.

Summary and Key Takeaways

This section of the chapter dived deep into the concept and discourse of effective shared decision making and how, in practice, this can be translated to develop a comprehensive and useful tool and/or intervention. The overall objective of shared decision-making is to improve overall health outcomes by improving the engagement of doctor–patient communication.

Concept	Guiding principles
Collaboration through communication	Good doctor–patient communication is essential to health promotion, disease prevention and a collaborative discussion.
Transparency of information	The information provided to individuals should be clear, understandable, accurate and readable with consideration of their health literacy ability
Informed choice	Information should be balanced and fair to enable informed choice
Empower and activation	Individuals feel in control and have the opportunities and self-efficacy to take action

As a reminder, the premise of shared decision making is built on the concepts below and some guiding principles discussed, as outlined in the table below.

Understanding and Measuring Behavioural Attributes When Developing Patient Engagement Strategies and Solutions

A behaviour attribute is described as an individual characteristic aligned with a number of factors, such as a personality trait, motivations, skills, and knowledge; this is often a good method for measuring individual behaviours.

Carl Jung believed that archetypes were models of people, behaviour or personalities. Inborn tendencies play a role in influencing human behaviour. He suggested that these models are innate, universal and hereditary. Archetypes are unlearned functions which help organise how we experience certain things. The actual way in which an archetype is expressed or realised depends upon a number of factors, including cultural influence and unique personal experiences (Vedor 2023).

When working in the patient engagement space, often the clients I work with across pharma are interested in learning more about specific behavioural attributes; gone are the days when solutions were developed based on a number of unidentifiable, unknown attributes (there was no real way to rationalise how the solution was targeting specific attributes). We now understand that the most effective solution is when there is an opportunity to personalise the journey. Personalisation can be effectively integrated only when there is a better understanding of specific attributes the solution is targeting (it may seem confusing, but there is logic).

In this chapter, I plan to discuss the process of attribute identification using case study scenarios in which I have implemented this approach in practice. In Chap. 2, I outlined some health psychology models that are useful, especially when you are trying to target the intervention.

To put this in to context, I will start by defining an example;

Scenario 1

Company E is working on asthma. People diagnosed with asthma have been living with this for a number of years, many since childhood. Therefore, the assumption is that patients are very informed about the method of managing asthma. Company E agrees to this consensus and understands that investing in developing interventions is probably not as helpful as there is so much material and information which exists, overloading people with more information is probably not the best or valuable for the patient community. However, company E would like to reach a specific audience within the patient population, those who are not activated and require support in managing their asthma.

How can they (1) identify the patient subtype they are trying to reach (2) what types of attributes of the individual do they need to consider and (3) what types of messaging and/or behaviour change techniques should they be building into their content and/or interventions?

The above-mentioned case scenario is one I have heard a few times over my years collaborating with pharma. Given that there is no one specific method for addressing the above challenge (brief), the method I am going to discuss is one that I have crafted through trial and error; hence, sharing my experience will hopefully help you structure what might work for you when faced with this brief.

Question 1: Identify the Patient Subtype the Project Will Target

Continuing with the therapy areas for asthma, we know that there are different types of asthma: allergic, seasonal, occupational and others, such as uncontrolled asthma and severe asthma. Identifying the type of asthma that the company would like to focus on is considered one variable for the subtype. Usually, the pharma team will have a focused area associated with the indication; for this example, let's say this is severe asthma.

Variable 1: Severe Asthma

What do we know about severe asthma? To answer this question, there is a need to complete some insight generation via a literature review or targeted research. However, what are you looking for in this research? The objective of insight generation will be to understand the disease experience of severe asthma patients to determine the typical behaviours advocated through this research. By doing so, it may be likely that you discover collective experiences that can be subdivided into groups. For the purpose of identifying asthma attributes, two types of severe asthma patients were found.

Variable 2: Subgroups: (1) Disengaged and Low Confidence and (2) Engaged, Not Action Oriented

The two subtypes provide a good foundation for starting to dive deeper into the key attributes. A description of the subtypes is provided below.

- ***Disengaged and low confidence:*** individuals in this group are passive, lack confidence, have low general knowledge, are not goal oriented and have poor adherence to treatment and/or doctor advice.
- ***Engaged, not action oriented:*** individuals have knowledge, but there are still knowledge gaps. Struggle to implement any planned action and often believe that this is not in their control.

Patient activation measures can be used within research if, during the subgroup identification process, there is capacity to develop a short quantitative study of the patient activation measure (PAM) developed by Insignia Health offered segmentation via a short questionnaire (Insignia Health Patient Activation).

Question 2: What Types of Attributes of the Subgroups Do You Need to Consider?

After the subgroups have been outlined above, the next step is to identify the attributes/cluster behaviours associated with each subgroup. This will support message targeting in the next stage. As a health psychologist, I would go somewhat further into the subgroups and would be interested in understanding other determinates of these groups: (1) psychological health, (2) illness perception, (3) medication necessity and (4) social support. There are measures that can support testing the determinates, as listed below:

1. ***Psychological health:*** Patient Health Questionnaire (PHQ-9—measures mood) and Generalised Anxiety Disorders Scale (GAD—measures anxiety).
2. ***Illness perception:*** Brief Illness Perception Questionnaire (B-IPQ)—eight item self-reported measure. Higher scores indicate a more negative illness perception.
3. ***Medication necessity:*** Necessity-concerns framework—the ability to assess relationships between two separate dimensions—patients' necessity beliefs and concerns about medication—two predictors that predict the outcome of nonadherence to medication (Horne and Weinman 1999).
4. ***Social support:*** A 12-item self-reported multidimensional scale of perceived social support (MSPSS) measures levels of social support (friends, family and significant others).

Capturing the above information about the subgroups will further enhance and deepen the understanding of how to target interventions for this group. Not to complicate matters, but at this point, having an interventional framework can support the transfer of subgroup determinates to behaviour change techniques using the behaviour change taxonomy COM-B. The authors are referring to the health psychology models in Chap. 2.

The COM-B helps shape the subgroups and the determinates into a structured scope, as outlined in the example below, to help illustrate this (Table 3.1).

The interpretation of the table above is outlined below, as is a reminder of the attribute we are building (this is a hypothetical example; the below is not based on real research but rather an illustration of how to turn insights into a tailored model to assign messaging):

Table 3.1 Summary of subgroups 1 and 2: determinants—structured within the COM-B

COM-B	Capabilities	Opportunities	Motivation	Necessity- concern about medication	Social support	Psychological health
G1: Disengaged and low confidence	***Psychological:*** low ***Physical:*** medium	***Physical:*** high ***Social:*** medium	*Reflective:* ***low*** *Automatic:* ***low***	***Necessity: low*** ***Concern: high***	Medium	Low
G2: Engaged and not action orientation	***Psychological:*** medium ***Physical:*** medium	***Physical:*** *high* ***Social:*** medium	*Reflective:* ***low*** *Automatic:* ***medium***	***Necessity: high*** ***Concern: low***	Medium	Low/medium

Therapy focus: Severe asthma

Group 1: Disengaged and had low confidence

Profile: Passive, lack confidence, low general knowledge, not goal-oriented and poor adherence to treatment and/or doctor advice.

Attribute type: This group has low psychological capability but high physical opportunity. The reflective and automatic motivation of these individuals is low, and beliefs associated with the necessity for treatment are low, while concerns about treatment are high. The social network and support of these individuals are considered medium (average range); however, their overall psychological health is low (which is likely contributing to their motivational drivers).

Group 2: Engaged and Not-action Orientation

Profile: Individuals have knowledge, but there are still knowledge gaps. Struggle to implement any planned action and often believe that this is not in their control.

Attribute type: This group, on average, is psychologically capable and has high opportunities (to access support and healthcare). The reflective motivation of these patients is low, their necessity for treatment is high (believe medication is necessary for disease management), and their overall medication concerns are low (not concerned about medication administration, usage or side effects). They have average social support, and their overall psychological health is manageable.

The profile summaries provided a holistic outline of the two groups, and the descriptions supported the overall targeting.

Question 3: What Types of Messaging and/or Behaviour Change Techniques Could Be Built in the Content and/or Intervention?

During this phase, the elements all come together, with reference to the behaviour taxonomy earlier; using this as a guide to start with the alignment is essential. There are, of course, other behaviour change techniques that can be incorporated into the matrix; therefore, there is no rule or process that requires a rigid framework. It is important that the spectrum of techniques be introduced and recommended to further enhance behavioural personalisation.

The tables below will provide example frameworks for how to incorporate behaviour change techniques and discussions across the matrix, as illustrated in the two examples below.

Summary of Subgroups 1 and 2: Determinants—Structured Within the COM-B and Targeted BCTs (Michie et al. 2011) (Tables 3.2 and 3.3)

The example behaviour change techniques outlined for groups 1 and 2 are focused on the areas across the matrix, which suggests that the group capacity was low and required further interventional messaging. Therefore, the grey-shaded area in the table aligns with what is being targeted with the behaviour change techniques. Although there are a number of BCTs within the taxonomy, 93, to be specific (Cane et al. 2015), it is helpful to read through each domain and BCT type to support the drafting of the descriptions, as you can use multiple of the same BCTs but in a different capacity, i.e., (1) BCT: Instructions on how to perform a behaviour (education domain), but the description can differ depending on the stakeholder the interventional plan is being devised for, healthcare professional, or patient the description of how your developing the messaging will differ.

As mentioned earlier, when utilising frameworks or matrices such as this one, it is always better to formulate a method that is comfortable and suitable for individual tasks to develop interventions.

Continuing with the illustration of embedding BCT into patient-facing content (which is where the majority of health psychologists focus on working across pharma initiatives), I will now build an example of how to move to the next level of implementation science.

Table 3.2 Group 1: Disengaged and low confidence: *example of behaviour change techniques and interventions recommended*

			Capabilities		**Opportunities**		**Motivation**	
BCT	**Function**	**Description**	*Physical*	*Psych*	*Social*	*Physical*	*Reflective*	*Automatic*
Instructions on how to perform the behaviour	Education	Patient material focused on how practical method to manage asthma						
Goal setting	Enablement	Clear SMART goals focused on asthma management						
Verbal persuasion about capabilities	Persuasion	Clear information on asthma management being success if actions is taken						
Focus on past success	Persuasion	Patients who have low engagement are reminder to be reflective on past health success						
Social reward	Incentivisation	Patients' goals are linked to personal and social rewards, i.e., Improved health provides a means to travel						

*BCT: behaviour change technique

Table 3.3 Group 2: Engaged and not-action orientation: *example of behaviour change techniques and interventions recommended*

			Capabilities		Opportunities		Motivation	
BCT	**Function**	**Description**	*Physical*	*Psych*	*Social*	*Physical*	*Reflecti ve*	*Automati c*
Self-monitoring	Enablement	Patients are provided with a self-management app/tracker to manage asthma experience						
Problem solving	Environment al restructure	Patients are provided with problem statements and frequently asked questions to dismay asthma myths						
Feeback on behaviour	Persuasion	Patients provided with a comparative patient story discussing impact and outcome						
Social reward	Incentivisati on	Patients are provided with positive reinforcement message, such as praise, recognition, attention, or acceptance, throughout patient material.						
Instruction on how to perform the behaviour	Education	Clarity on how to implement and action plan for day-to-day asthma management						

*BCT: behaviour change technique

Turning Behaviour Change Techniques into Content Messaging

I am often asked, What happens now? We understand the patient subgroups we are targeting and have aligned the behaviour change techniques; what does this mean?

The next step is the exciting part; this is when you can start to actually see the recommendation coming to life. For the purposes of this example, we can assume that the client (pharma) has decided that for group 1, they would like to develop a consultation guide for healthcare professionals, and for group 2, the focus will be a patient support website.

- Solution 1: Healthcare discussion guide (Table 3.4)
- Solution 2: Patient support website (Table 3.5)

Table 3.4 Group 1: Solution 1 blueprint

BCT	Function	Description	Patient support material
Instructions on how to perform the behaviour	Education	Patient material focused on how practical method to manage asthma	Topic 1: Living with Asthma
Goal setting	Enablement	Clear SMART goals focused on asthma management	SMART goal setting and action planning guidelines
Verbal persuasion about capabilities	Persuasion	Clear information on asthma management/success if actions is taken	Positive-gain message framing narratives—emphasis of health outcomes if adherent to treatment
Focus on past success	Persuasion	Patients who have low engagement are reminder to be reflective on past health success	Patient case studies—peer to peer examples across the community can be good examples of success
Social reward	Incentivisation	Patients' goals are linked to personal and social rewards, i.e., Improved health provides a means to travel	Patient storytelling examples through patient videos

Table 3.5 Group 2: Solution 2

BCT	Function	Description	Healthcare professional discussion guide
Self-monitoring	Enablement	Patients are provided with a self-management app/tracker to manage asthma experience	Mobile/web assisted patient support programme
Problem solving	Environmental restructure	Patients are provided with problem statements and frequently asked questions to dismay asthma myths	Myth buster—frequently asked questions module
Feeback on behaviour	Persuasion	Patients provided with a comparative patient story discussing impact and outcome	Patient videos—peers to peer connectively
Social reward	Incentivisation	Patients are provided with positive reinforcement message, such as praise, recognition, attention, or acceptance, throughout patient material.	Positive-gain messaging
Instruction on how to perform the behaviour	Education	Clarity on how to implement and action plan for day-to-day asthma management	How to video: treatment administration, planning a day out, tracking pollen count

Decision-Making and Message Framing: What Does This Mean?

Prospect theory was developed by economists Daniel Kahneman and Amos Tversky in 1979. The theory discusses the psychological explanation of the process executed in the method of decision-making and, more importantly, how an individual is able to cognitively, emotionally and rationally balance risk through decision-making. The model attempts to explain the process of decision-making; one of the important assumptions of this model is that the way a decision is framed influences the individual in the decisional process. Tversky and Kahneman (1987) stated that "*the prospect theory holds that individuals are more influenced by the possibility of a loss than the prospect of an equivalent gain.*"

In terms of the concept and associations of health decisions, which are significantly more risky, theory suggests that the method in which health information is framed for the general public can contribute to how individuals might respond to it. This is why I found this theory an important one to discuss in this section. Often, in healthcare communication, people are unconscious about how context and the way words are written and, at times, are required to have conscious reactions to health information or when they have been left with a key decision to make about their health, i.e., about preventative screening, treatment choice and vaccinations; these are just a few examples. In such circumstances, individuals will balance the "gain" and/or "loss" of the actions that trigger the decision and pathway they take. Gisbert-Perez et al. (2022) performed a systematic review of prospect theory and identified three main attributes of prospect theory in healthcare. (1) Prospect theory indicates that people will act differently depending on whether a situation is gain- or loss-framed compared to other situations. (2) The situation may have an impact on preventive health behaviour and the actions of that individual, i.e., vaccination or invasive screening; when the risk is immediate or negative, such as pain, it is considered greater than the potential gain, i.e., screening will detect any cancerous cells early. (3) The theory predicts that reframing health outcomes with respect to certainty would change decisions about health behaviours (as there is often an overweighting certainty). Essentially, the research emphasised that in the healthcare context, "gain frames" are likely to be more beneficial when promoting preventative health information. Importantly, the model predicts that people will be more likely to take risks when they are experiencing losses than when they are experiencing gains.

The utilisation of the prospect theory framework can significantly support and enable health-related messaging development by communication healthcare agencies and public health organisations to optimise the framing of the messaging to activate individuals and increase engagement.

Pharma companies are developing a number of disease awareness campaigns, branded treatment information, healthcare professionals' consultation guides, advertisements and external posters with the purpose of helping individuals make key decisions about their healthcare. What this theory tells us is that using a

Table 3.6 Message framing examples

Positive "gains frame"	Negative "loss frame"
Eating a balanced diet has several health benefits and reduces the chances of developing health problems.	Eating unhealthy food will increase your chances of obesity and other health problems such as cholesterol and type 2 diabetes.
Doctor tells a patient the procedure has a 90% success rate	Doctor tells patients there is a 10% chance of the procedure failing
That drink is 90% sugar free	That drink is 10% sugar

"framing" method should elicit engagement and personalise the messaging based on how one would assess a "loss and gain". Gallagher and Updegraff (2011) emphasised that "*how a health message is framed is an important consideration in designing messages that promote preventive behaviours*". However, it is important to be mindful that the process of decision making is based on other external attributes that should be considered, such as past experiences, current circumstances, cultural norms and individual preferences (Tversky and Kahneman 1973).

Therefore, what does messaging framing actually mean? Well-to-put this into context, I have outlined some examples of how to develop messages with the emphasis of gain/positive framing vs. loss/negative framing (Table 3.6).

Gallagher and Updegraff (2012) found that gain-framed messages were more likely to encourage and promote behaviour than loss-framed messages were. The cognitive bias associated with this process is that individuals' choices are influenced by the information presented to them, irrespective of the substance of the message. As mentioned earlier, message framing is often used in health communication messages and promotion/prevention campaigns.

References

Cane J, Richardson M, Johnston M, Ladha R, Michie S (2015) From lists of behaviour change techniques (BCTs) to structured hierarchies: comparison of two methods of developing a hierarchy of BCTs. Br J Health Psychol 20(1):130–150. https://doi.org/10.1111/bjhp.12102. Epub 2014 May 12

Cyril S, Smith BJ, Renzaho AMN (2016) Systematic review of empowerment measures in health promotion. Health Promot Int 31(4):809–826. https://doi.org/10.1093/heapro/dav059

Dewalt DA, Berkman ND, Sheridan S, Lohr KN, Pignone MP (2004) Literacy and health outcomes: a systematic review of the literature. J Gen Intern Med 19(12):1228–1239. https://doi.org/10.1111/j.1525-1497.2004.40153.x. PMID:15610334; PMCID: PMC1492599

Edgman-Levitan S, Schoenbaum SC (2021) Patient-centred care: achieving higher quality by designing care through the patient's eyes. Isr J Health Policy Res 10(1):21. https://doi.org/10.1186/s13584-021-00459-9. PMID: 33673875; PMCID: PMC7934513

Gallagher KM, Updegraff JA (2011) When 'fit' leads to fit, and when 'fit' leads to fat: how message framing and intrinsic vs. extrinsic exercise outcomes interact in promoting physical activity. Psychol Health 26:819–834. https://doi.org/10.1080/08870446.2010.505983

Gallagher KM, Updegraff JA (2012) Health message framing effects on attitudes, intentions, and behavior: a meta-analytic review. Ann Behav Med 43(1):101–116. https://doi.org/10.1007/s12160-011-9308-7. Erratum in: Ann Behav Med. 2013 Aug;46(1):127

General Medical Council (1999) Seeking patients' consent: the ethical considerations. General Medical Council, London

Gisbert-Pérez J, Martí-Vilar M, González-Sala F (2022) Prospect theory: a bibliometric and systematic review in the categories of psychology in web of science. Healthcare (Basel) 10(10):2098. https://doi.org/10.3390/healthcare10102098. PMID: 36292546; PMCID: PMC9601776

Horne R, Weinman J (1999) Patients' beliefs about prescribed medicines and their role in adherence to treatment in chronic physical illness. J Psychosom Res 47:555–567. https://doi.org/10.1016/S0022-3999(99)00057-4

Insignia Health Patient Activation Measure (PAM) Survey levels. Available from http://www.insigniahealth.com/products/pam-survey

Kahneman D, Tversky A (1979) Prospect theory: an analysis of decision under risk. Econometría 47:263–292. https://doi.org/10.2307/1914185

Kim K, Lee S (2016) Psychological empowerment. Last reviewed: 21 September 2020, last modified: 28 April 2016. https://doi.org/10.1093/OBO/9780199846740-0090

Marteau TM, Dormandy E, Michie S (2001) A measure of informed choice. Health Expect 4(2):99–108. https://doi.org/10.1046/j.1369-6513.2001.00140.x. PMID: 11359540; PMCID: PMC5060053

Michie S, van Stralen MM, West R (2011) The behaviour change wheel: a new method for characterising and designing behaviour change interventions. Implement Sci 6:42. https://doi.org/10.1186/1748-5908-6-42. PMID: 21513547; PMCID: PMC3096582.

Nutbeam D (2000) Health literacy as a public health goal: a challenge for contemporary health education and communication strategies into the 21st Century. Health Promot Int 15:259–267

Nutbeam D (2009) Defining and measuring health literacy: what can we learn from literacy studies? Int J Public Health 54:303–305. https://doi.org/10.1007/s00038-009-0050-x

Paasche-Orlow MK, Parker RM, Gazmararian JA et al (2005) The prevalence of limited health literacy. J Gen Intern Med 20:175–184. https://doi.org/10.1111/j.1525-1497.2005.40245.x

Stacey D, Légaré F, Lewis KB, Barry MJ, Bennett CL, Eden KB, Holmes-Rovner M, Llewellyn-Thomas H, Lyddiatt A, Thomson RG, Trevena LJ (2017) Decision aids for people facing health treatment or screening decisions. Cochrane Database Syst Rev 4:CD001431

Tversky A, Kahneman D (1973) Judgment under uncertainty: Heuristics and biases. Oregon Research Inst., Vol. 13(1).

Tversky A, Kahneman D (1987) Rational choice and the framing of decisions. In: Hogarth RM, Reder MW (eds) Rational choice: the contrast between economics and psychology. University of Chicago Press, Chicago, pp 67–94

Vedor JE (2023) Revisiting Carl Jung's archetype theory a psychobiological approach. Biosystems 234:105059. ISSN 0303-2647

Chapter 4
Case Studies in Practice-Collobration: Pharmaceutical Professionals Who Have Collaborated with Psychologists

Often, a question I am asked is whether there are any case studies or example projects that demonstrate how a health psychologist has contributed to and/or developed a patient engagement solution in partnership with a pharmaceutical company. Well you are in luck.

In this chapter, I will describe project case studies, all of which are fictional; of course, I need to be mindful that the identities of the companies I work with are protected. Nonetheless, I will provide a 360° perspective of the approach I utilise, which often always starts with "the brief", strategically moves to the "process/method" and, finally, the "solution/delivery."

Before diving deep into the case studies, I wanted to provide you with some insight into the spectrum of projects a health psychology team has worked across; by no means is this an endless list, but a thoughtful overview of the depth of the transferrable skills learned in the health psychology doctorate has absolutely come in handy.

- **Patient experience mapping: understanding the lived experience of patients/caregivers.**
- **Psychological intervention for patients/caregivers/family members.**
- **Behaviour change modelling: Patient segmentation/patient activation.**
- Shared decision-making and decision-making tools for healthcare professionals.
- Health literacy and health promotion.

S. Riaz, *Patient Engagement in Pharma*,
https://doi.org/10.1007/978-3-031-56340-9_4

Patient Study 1: Patient Experience Mapping: Understanding the Emotional and Clinical Patient Journey

Project Brief: What Is This Approach?

Patient experience mapping is a method for illustrating a comprehensive picture of a patient's journey and lived experiences across a specific condition. There are many different iterations of how a patient journey map can be developed or presented across disciplines. The example methodology I will discuss is one that relates to the approach I have often used as a health psychologist.

Why Do Pharma Companies Commission This Work?

There may be a number of reasons why a pharma company commits to a patient journey map; this can be introduced at any specific time point throughout the product development journey. Some may want to understand the patients' lived experience prelaunch (product is still in clinical phase development); therefore, pharma teams are keen to start creating an insight base about the patients' experience to determine how this new drug will enter the journey. Will it meet a specific or range of unmet needs identified across the journey? What is this product solving for the patient? In addition, a patient journey may be initiated at postlaunch, the product has been on the market for a year or more, and the brand team (pharma teams aligned with the product) is interested in determining whether there have been any changes to the patient experience or if there are any specific challenges or barriers impacting the patient experience related to the product or condition. Below is an example of this in practice:

Scenario one: Company A is launching a new treatment for a rare disease; therefore, the existing research on this disease is minimal. There is a need to dive deeper into understanding the lived experience of this condition and explore the perspectives of healthcare professionals.

Scenario two: The Company B product has been on the market for 2 years; however, healthcare professionals have identified a number of adherence challenges, and patients are not staying on treatment for more than 3 months. Therefore, there is a need to explore the challenges associated with treatment and disease experience.

Methodology: How Can You Scope Research Design to Fulfil This Objective?

There is no way or method to complete a patient journey mapping project. However, over the years, I have learned to use an approach that is not linear but dynamic based on the level of existing research available. The majority of the time, pharma teams will have completed some type of research for the specific disease area of interest. It is helpful to start here with a data immersion/audit phase. However, the audit was not just completed via a traditional linear approach. Using a psychological model as a template to complete an audit enables a comprehensive analysis of existing research and outlines where data gaps may exist. When recommending further qualitative or quantitative research, a more targeted approach to the semi-structured interview guide should be provided.

Once the data immersion phase is complete and the qualitative discussion guide is formalised, a one-to-one interview with those diagnosed with the condition and caregivers/family members living with the individual diagnosed and healthcare professionals specialising in this field provides a 360° perspective of the lived experience across the treatment/disease journey. The final step is the analysis and interpretation of the data before turning this into an illustrative journey to demonstrate the lived experience.

How Can a Psychologist Contribute to This Analysis?

Psychologists go through years of learning how to interpret qualitative and quantitative data, as with other disciplines, such as psychology. However, a psychologist trained to work therapeutically with people is able to take narratives and dive beyond just surface-level interpretation. They are able to formulate a thematic analysis and interpretation of the experience and holistically find similarities and differences in those experiences without losing the uniqueness of individual experiences. From my experience, this approach can work in a few steps:

- Step 1: Transcribe the interview.
- Step 2: Review the transcripts in stages to determine the key experiences per stage of the journey, i.e., pre-diagnosis, diagnosis, treatment and ongoing management (living with). (I usually develop a separate doc/excel sheet to capture key experiences across the five journey stages, constructing an analysis framework.)
- Step 3: Once you have gone through all of the interview transcripts and extracted the insights into the analysis framework, you have to reanalyse the data within the framework to formulate a populational analysis of the research sample.

- Step 4: Developing the patient journey framework: using the populational analysis data, you start to construct the journey, which now has the segmentations of insights plotted across the key stages.
- Step 5: Making the journey useful for pharma teams (this piece of work is not just a research project), you have to make it applicable and valuable to the commissioning party, who in this instance is the pharmaceutical company (this is why using health psychology models is helpful). At this stage, the insights across the journey need to be clear and comprehensive to align with the overall commercial and research objectives set out by the commissioning team. The questions I have often come across are as follows: *How are these data useful for us? What can they do to improve the experience and support patients require?* What are the unmet needs and gaps in services for patients, caregivers and healthcare professionals? To do this effectively, I recommend ensuring that there is alignment with the strategic imperatives developed by the pharma team (I usually describe strategic imperatives as "main themes" for pharma teams to consider). Strategic imperatives will support guiding and developing a patient engagement strategy for a specific disease area (as discussed in earlier chapters on how to develop an effective patient engagement strategy).
- Final step: Making the journey stand out and actionable: The importance of the journey is to make it actionable and enable pharma teams to implement tactics to support and improve the patient experience. However, remember, no one has time to read pages and pages of insights and interpretation. Therefore, it is imperative that you bring some creativity and craft to the final patient journey. My personal rule is to ensure that the comprehensiveness of the journey is valued and not compromised; therefore, an illustrative "landing page" of the journey demonstrating the experience and flow of the patient group will provide a good summary before readers dive deeper into specific stage summaries. The landing page works well if it includes interactive features to the design, such as pop-out boxes, % icons, and clickable content boxes, which lead to stage summary pages, videos or audio narratives (if consent is obtained by the interviewees) across the journey to bring the experience to life.

Reflection as a Health Psychologist

I have contributed to and worked on a number of patient journey projects over the last 10 years for a number of pharmaceutical teams and companies. The approach I have described is one that I often utilised as my foundational framework. The holisticness of this method fits within an objective or challenge provided to me by industry. When I first started to work in this field, I quickly realised that there was no set method that I could lift and use; I had to create one that made sense to work with for myself and the team as we were trying to establish something that could be versatile and applicable. One of the skills of a psychologist is to diversify the models used to formulate and interpret lived experiences, leveraging and bridging existing qualitative analysis methods such as thematic analysis, interpretive phenomenological analysis (IPA), grounded theory, ethnography and case studies to personalise the interpretation appropriate for patient journey flow. Studying research methods through the entire journey of becoming a psychologist truly supported my ability to leverage the parts of different methods. The second reflection, as mentioned earlier, involved the skills learned to interpret the narratives of the patient groups further and then surface-level insights; it was not just describing what people said in the interview but also how to collate those experiences, create cluster themes and describe that experience (in other words, not just state the facts, provide an interpretation or story) to take the reader on that journey. A psychologist often completes in-depth interpretations of lived experiences to develop therapeutic or interventional plans of action; therefore, those skills can be leveraged here, which I found to be an added benefit for the end result.

Case Study 2: Psychological Intervention for Patients/Caregivers/Family Members

Project Brief: What Is This Approach?

Psychological interventions are those directed to elicit change or provide therapeutic support to those who require it. The development of psychological interventions is usually triggered when there is an identified unmet need for the patient group. These types of interventions can be preventative, therapeutic or focused on behavioural change. The objective of the intervention will be specific and based on the overall focus.

Why Do Pharma Companies Commission This Work?

Pharma companies often develop patient support programmes or initiatives to support patients across a number of identified needs or support gaps, especially if the current healthcare services are not offering support or if there is a long waiting time for patients to access support. Traditionally and currently, pharma companies lead in developing patient material to support patients in (1) learning about their diagnosis, (2) providing treatment information, (3) providing support services and/or patient groups that patients can access, and (4) providing lifestyle information. (5) Symptom tracker/appointment reminders (this is not an exhaustive list but a top-line example of types of information and support offered by companies). However, over the years, there has been a significant need to support patients/caregivers/family members across their psychological wellbeing; similarly, healthcare professionals are identifying the lack of services to which they can refer their patients. With this dilemma of support needs vs lack of services, pharma companies are moving into offering low-intensity, psychoeducational support to those who need it via patient support solutions. However, to do this right, there is a drive for psychologists to support this initiative. Below are two scenarios in which this type of work involves commissioning:

In scenario one, Company A identified through primary market research that there is a significant unmet psychological need for patients diagnosed with metastatic cancer. The current wait time for support is 7–12 months. Similarly, family members and caregivers supporting patients have expressed a need for psychological support.

Scenario two: Company B carried out a survey with healthcare professionals working in paediatric care. The treatment offered by this company is administered via an injection; however, there is an identified barrier that impacts parents and professionals when administering treatment. Children are significantly reluctant, and some have developed a needle phobia.

Methodology: How Do You Fulfil This Objective?

One of the major professional competencies in psychology is researching, designing and developing psychological interventions. There is no one way of proposing how to design an effective psychological intervention; what I am going to describe is the method I have adapted and used when working with pharma companies that offer patient support solutions via a digital platform. Therefore, the type of intervention I will discuss is offered digitally and self-directed by the audience for which it was developed.

Step 1: Do your research: understand the audience you are developing this intervention for, specifically the subtypes and attributes of the group (attributes also referred to as persona types). If we take scenario one into consideration, metastatic cancer patients' quality of life and disease burden will differ from those of early-stage cancer patients; therefore, factoring this difference is important when considering the tone and language incorporated into the intervention. Similarly, in scenario two, the paediatric patient's user experience will differ, and consideration of how the intervention will be delivered is important, e.g., animated content, interactive features, gamification elements, and reward incentives.

Step 2: Try not to overwhelm the interventional design: When developing an intervention, you might be tempted to include everything to ensure that it is applicable to everyone and everything. The importance of remembering quality over quantity is appreciated, especially when the audience is already overwhelmed with managing their disease impact.

Step 3: Choose a therapeutic model: psychological interventions work well when they are founded on a therapeutic model. For example, cognitive behavioural therapy included acceptance commitment therapy (ACT), mindfulness therapy, and rational motive behaviour therapy (REBT). Depending on the type of outcome you are measuring, using one of the preexisting models will help to frame the psychological intervention and develop low-intensity, self-directed sessions.

Step 4: Cocreate and validate the psychological solution: One of the musts I have learned over the years is to cocreate and validate the idea with the audience, who will be the ones using the solution. By testing it with this group, you will be able to obtain valuable feedback and recommendations to improve the solution; additionally, testing of tone, design and execution will be performed.

Step 5: Find an expert in this field: I have observed from personal experience that experts are not always offered the opportunity to develop solutions. I am a firm believer that to do this right, finding a psychologist to write the content for the psychological intervention will help to ensure that the direction is appropriate. For example, if the decision is to develop a low-intensity CBT digital solution for patients living with metastatic cancer, a trained psychologist will understand how to segment the sessions and the type/level of content that is manageable. To put this into context, below is an example of a low-intensity CBT digital solution:

Example of psychological modules includes within a patient support solution

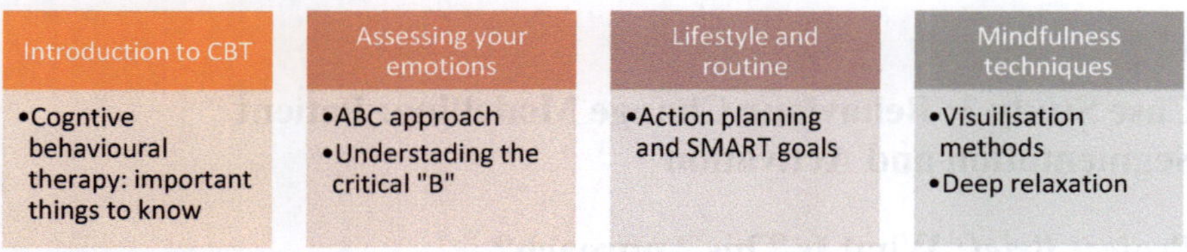

Step 6: Measure the outcome and impact: With any type of intervention, the indicators of success and usefulness are determined by measuring the outcome. Including patient-reported outcome opportunities within the solution is key. For example, you can include a quality-of-life questionnaire at the start of the intervention, asking participants to complete this questionnaire prior to beginning, which can be repeated at the end of the intervention to determine if any change in quality of life is captured. As it is a digital solution, there are other options for metrics that can be included, i.e., the number of visits to each session, the time needed to complete a session, and per session feedback. Collecting digital non-health analytics can also be useful indicators of intervention success.

Reflection as a Health Psychologist

During my doctorate training, I was exposed to different types of behavioural and psychological preventative interventions. I also found this content module interesting and one I immensely enjoyed. Developing something that was actually going to make a change was exciting and one of the reasons why I studied health psychology.

Traditionally, pharma companies have not developed such interventions as mentioned earlier; however, to date, based on my personal experience, I have supported the development of many psychoeducational and interventional solutions that have been delivered globally and translated into many languages. This is a good indicator that there is a need to offer psychological support solutions, especially when the service offered via the NHS is limited because capacity and private therapy can be costly and unaffordable for many individuals. There is a great opportunity for pharma to support developing services such as emotional support, but with the caveat of ensuring that solutions such as this are developed by trained professionals who understand the sensitivity of those experiencing mental health challenges and can ensure that the language, content and purpose of the intervention are appropriate for the audience. When I first started to work in this space, there was no set blueprint for how to develop a digital psychological support solution while considering compliance and industry ethical considerations. Over the years, my experience has enabled me to craft the methodological flow outlined above, and working with different pharmaceutical companies always ensures that you are aware of their compliance and medical signs (for those who have experience in this field, I understand that this requires its own dedicated chapter).

Case Study 3: Behaviour Change Modelling: Patient Segmentation and Activation

Project Brief: What Is This Approach?

You may be familiar with the words, segmentation and activation. I have used these terms interchangeably throughout this book. For this final case study, I will discuss why patient segmentation and activation have become an area of interest for pharma companies and what interpretation these concepts are used across industries. For several years, psychologists have been learning about the art of human behaviour, personality traits, motivational drivers, barriers and enablers of engagement, decisional processes (why and how people make decisions), rational and irrational thought processes, etc. Recently, pharma teams have edged onto this concept and have started to learn how embracing these concepts can support them in supporting patients and healthcare professionals in engaging with the healthcare system, disease management and treatment adherence more effectively.

Why Do Pharma Companies Commission This Work?

Understanding human behaviour, or behavioural science, is an interesting and complex topic. Many have varied interpretations of what this means and its implementation. My reference to behaviour science and human behaviour is centred on my understanding as a psychologist. I often explain to others that we base our decisions on what we have experienced before in life, an analogy I often use to describe this as an "invisible handbag/bag/rucksack/briefcase" whatever makes sense for you. From an early age, this invisible bag stays with us, and as we experience events, view our environment, share interactions with family, friends and have good or difficult experiences, we collate them in our invisible bag. When we are then faced with similar situations, we lean to our invisible bag to analyse how to cope or react to the situation; sometimes we may not have preexisting experiences; therefore, we have to learn how to cope on the spot, which may be maladaptive or unhealthy. Other times, we find solutions to the situation as we had faced it prior, or someone in our environment had and we learn from that (these could have been healthy or unhealthy solutions). These experiences stay with us and form habits of "coping". Ultimately, every individual diagnosed with a health condition will address it uniquely, based on the contents of their invisible bag. Pharma companies are beginning to understand the notion that "one size does not fit all"; therefore, personalisation and segmentation were born out of the conclusion that any solutions offered to people require a form of flexibility rather than rigidity. Equally, every solution requires an "activated" individual who is willing to break old "habits" and learn different methods of engaging with services while considering their invisible bag. However, it is important to understand that individuals can still effectively engage with individuals who are not activated by personalising the solution to the level of activation they are comfortable with and teaching them to dispute unhealthy experiences to form new coping methods to manage comfortable situations. Let me explain this with some content:

Scenario one: Company A has been working on respiratory treatment for many years but has recently realised that patients are not adhering to their preventative medication. They would like to understand how to target information and messaging to those who are (1) activated in their treatment adherence or (2) not activated in treatment management; however, they understand that the messaging will have to be bespoke for both subgroups.

Scenario two: Company B has identified that their clinical trial participants are not diverse; for those who do engage, the retention is low (considerable percentage of dropout after 3 months), and the duration of the trial is 12 months. They are struggling to understand why they are not recruiting diverse populations for clinical trials, nor are they trying to understand the barriers or enablers of engagement and retention experienced by their potential study population.

Methodology: How Do You Fulfil This Objective?

Behaviour science is often associated with theories such as "nudge theory", which is applicable in advertisement messaging, healthcare preventative campaigns and, more prominently, the transtheoretical model (stages of change), which I have explained in detail in Chap. 2. Recently, the COM-B model and behaviour change taxonomy have taken precedence for psychologists who are developing preventative interventions via various channels. When I have been presented with the above two scenarios, I usually default to combining a number of health psychology theories and models that provide me with a wider scope to answer the challenge. There is no rule suggesting that combination approaches are incorrect; in fact, in counselling and therapeutic psychology, there are many modalities of therapy that are combined to provide the client with flexibility based on their needs. I have leaned on this flexible approach and often explore how best a combination of models can support the project scope set out by the pharmaceutical company. To answer the above two questions, below is the approach I often consider:

Step 1: Understand that the audience will support segmentation/grouping: Data immersion in existing research in a specific disease area and audience, including a targeted literature review on understanding the barriers and enablers of engagement (beliefs, perceptions, medication concerns), will help to formulate a foundational understanding of the overall experience.

Step 2: Choose your health psychology models: This is an important part, as it will support you in starting the segmentation of the data. For example, in scenario A, I may choose the stages of change model because it provides a structure across 5 activation stages (precontemplation, contemplation, preparation, action and maintenance). Using this structure, I can start to identify the types of factors that influence people to remain in stages 1–5 and what is required to move them to the next stage.

For scenario B, I might choose the COM-B model (description of this is in Chap. 2). The structure and factors associated with this model will support me in segmenting the data based on the population's capabilities, opportunities and motivation to elicit a behavioural change.

Step 3: Identify the behaviour change techniques/messaging: At this stage, the data are segmented into the appropriate factors, providing a holistic overview of where the challenges and unmet needs are. Along these lines, personas will have formed to support the alignment of the behaviour change techniques per segment.

Step 4: Develop the tactics and recommendations: This is the final blueprint for segmentation provided to the research commissioning team (pharma client). The model should include (1) segmentation groups, (2) behaviour change techniques/messaging per group, and (3) tactical interventions per segment to move people to become more activated across the activation spectrum.

Reflection as a Health Psychologist

Understanding behavioural attributes and designing solutions that align with these attributes will ensure that any patient material or intervention is available for the targeted audience. Returning to the notion that "one size does not fit all", we need to ensure that the project methods are flexible in how they are developed, allowing for content to be appropriate for people who are not as active in managing their healthcare journey (or may choose not to be) versus those who are activated. The content of the latter group, as mentioned earlier, differs, and this is how personalisation plays a part.

As a health psychologist, you are always determined to ensure that support is tailored, diverse and inclusive from a populational perspective. I have learned that using the method described within this case study enables you to target appropriately and measure outcomes. This is a trial and tested method, a good foundation to begin your journey of personalisation, but please remember, this is not a rigid, linear way of approaching segmentation. You may have your own preferences on how to create segments and may decide on some aspects of what is outlined to build upon your existing methods. Psychologists strive to elevate individual differences, but when working with pharma teams, there is a need to consider individual differences, elevate them to actional outcomes and deliver tactics across a number of populations.

Chapter 5
Key Considerations and Future Directions of Patient Engagement, Behaviour Science, Ethical Considerations and Further Training for Psychologist

Patient engagement is changing dynamically, as discussed throughout the chapters, and understanding how to effectively engage with patients while also developing bespoke solutions across all stakeholders is still evolving. There are a number of best practices introduced by psychologists, strategists, and researchers across the healthcare industry and effective solutions developed in partnership with the pharmaceutical industry. However, the establishment of psychologists engaging within this field is very new; despite the significant benefits of a health psychologist working with pharma, many people do not even know that this opportunity exists because it is not a pathway discussed openly in university or during training. As mentioned earlier, most health psychologists follow the traditional pathway of clinical practice, academics or research (including public health). However, working in a strategic, solution-focused capacity across the development of a product (medicine) globally is not thought of as an option, although the possibilities are there, people are not subjected to the opportunities.

The importance of patient engagement follows the guiding rules associated with one objective: improving outcomes (health, wellbeing, quality of life, disease, treatment and many others). Establishing a shared understanding of patient preferences through effective healthcare communication offers patients opportunities to discuss what matters to them. By encouraging active participation, the results can be efficacious for all patients, healthcare professionals, healthcare systems and overall economic outcomes, i.e., reduced healthcare costs and hospital readmissions.

Despite the awareness and elevated importance of effective patient engagement, there are still a number of barriers and challenges, particularly when considering future planning and direction. Accessing healthcare is still a significant hurdle; if access is limited, patients' opportunities to engage with their healthcare services are challenging. Cultural differences and language are still barriers to effective patient engagement; services are often not bespoke, and some patients find it challenging to adapt to ambiguous processes and pathways in healthcare. There is a need to introduce additional health literacy interventions and user-friendly technological

S. Riaz, *Patient Engagement in Pharma*,
https://doi.org/10.1007/978-3-031-56340-9_5

solutions. With the ongoing discussion centres on artificial intelligence (AI) and the drive to develop more innovative digital solutions, ensuring that patient data are protected is still unclear. I do want to emphasise that the evolution of digital solutions will take place, and moving with the times is important. There are many beneficial digital solutions that can be helpful for patients, such as side effects management tools (providing instance feedback or connectively to a healthcare provider if side effects are experienced), digital psychological programmes (accessing low-intensity emotional support, which is self-managed), personalised medicines, telehealth, virtual care and others. While digital tools are expanding, providing clear guidelines and developing protocols to ensure patient safety are highly important.

Other areas of consideration include the increase in patient advocacy engagement directly with pharma companies. These two types of engagement are positively associated with each other and discussed earlier; however, every company and patient organisation engage differently. By developing clear processes of engagement, ensuring that conflict is managed across organisations, making transparency of engagement is publicly available for the patient community to access and developing a consistent environment for all pharma and patient organisations to adhere to, it is imperative to move forward. Fostering change to ensure that engagement is dynamic, industry offers patient-centric opportunities, and future development is fostered in ethical technology with the aim of improving overall patient outcomes is a joint consensus appreciated by all.

As patients become more empowered in the decisions associated with their health, healthcare professionals are learning to adapt to the different patient segments/personalities and activation needs presented. This is where health psychology can be helpful. The models and techniques discussed within this book have been trialled and tested across solutions developed in collaboration with pharma companies. Historical models that emphasise doctor–patient communication, shared decision making, patient activation, message reframing and others, as well as techniques known and taught to health psychologists, can contribute significantly to industry-identified challenges they know exist across their patient's experience. However, I believe that there is a disconnect and gap in training psychologists to understand the drug development process, the structure of pharmaceutical companies, compliance and regulatory guidelines associated with developing and/or working with patients, and healthcare professionals across projects funded by pharmaceutical companies, developing strategic guidance and recommending opportunities to improve patient access and experience.

Despite this, the future of patient engagement is accelerating at a fast pace, establishing links through behaviour science and psychology, providing an evidence-based foundation for any patient solution initiated, providing a mechanism of measurement—which, for those who work across industries, knows and understands the importance of outcomes and measurements for demonstrating value, success measures and future investment.

Index

S. Riaz, *Patient Engagement in Pharma*,
https://doi.org/10.1007/978-3-031-56340-9

MIX
Papier aus verantwortungsvollen Quellen
Paper from responsible sources
FSC® C105338

If you have any concerns about our products,
you can contact us on
ProductSafety@springernature.com

In case Publisher is established outside the EU,
the EU authorized representative is:
Springer Nature Customer Service Center GmbH
Europaplatz 3, 69115 Heidelberg, Germany

Printed by Libri Plureos GmbH
in Hamburg, Germany